Novel Aspects on Motor Neuron Disease

Edited by Humberto Foyaca Sibat and Lourdes de Fátima Ibañez-Valdés

Published in London, United Kingdom

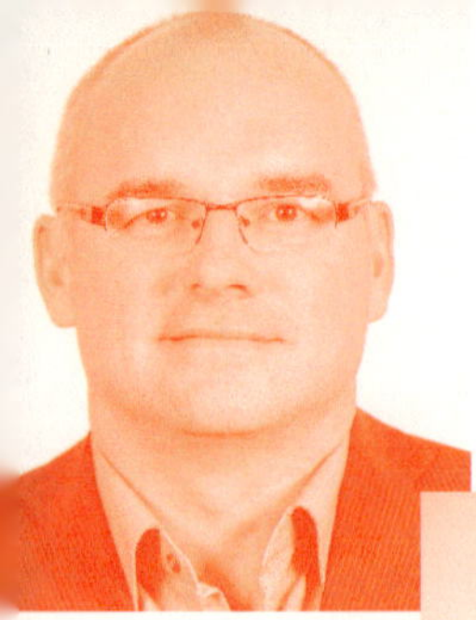
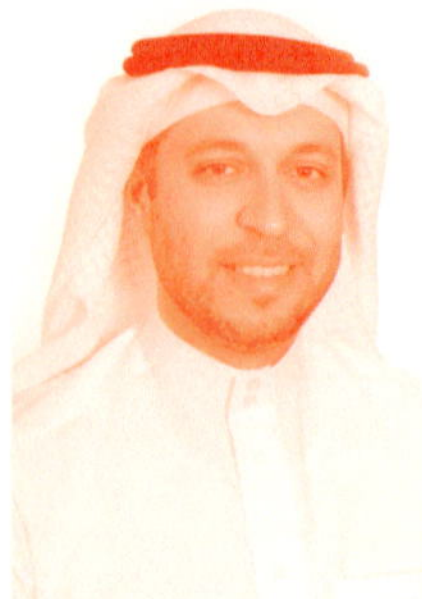
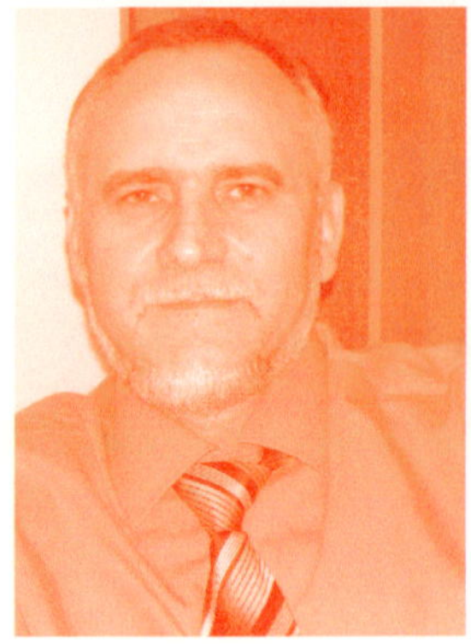
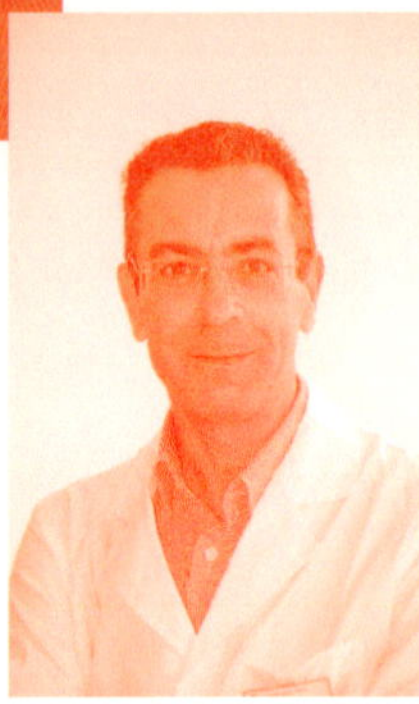
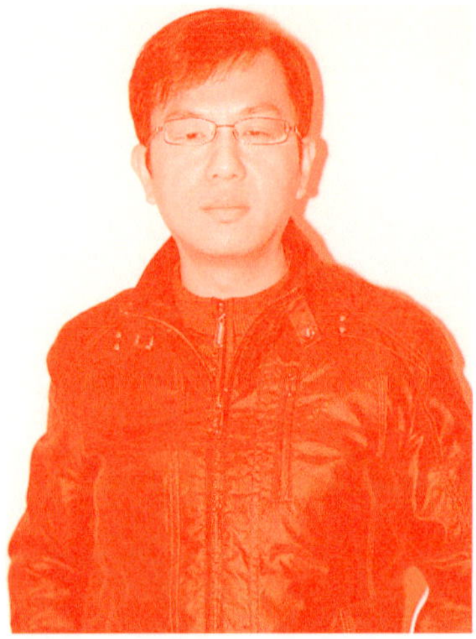
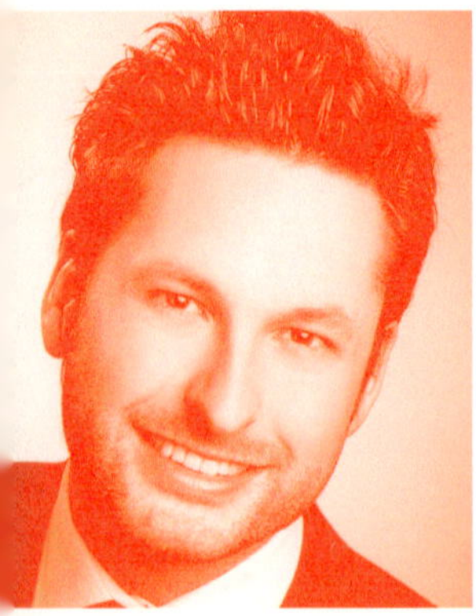
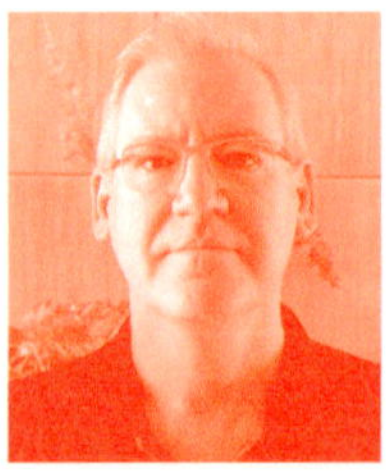

IntechOpen

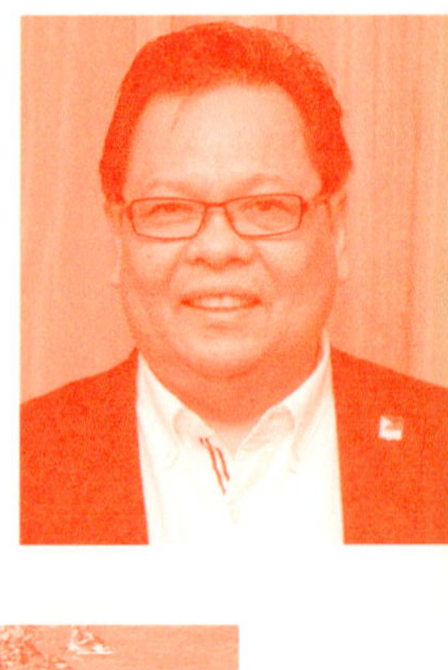
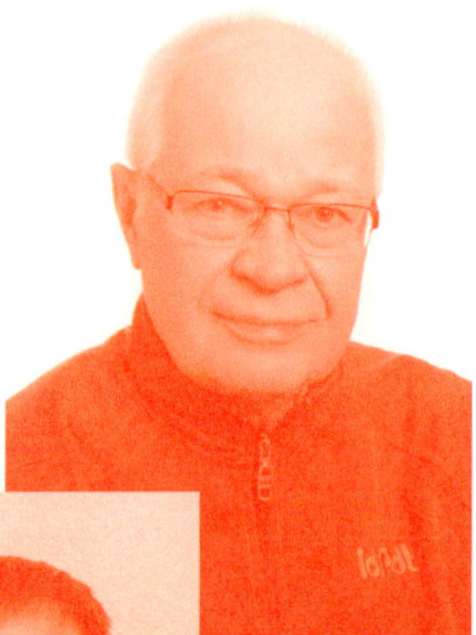
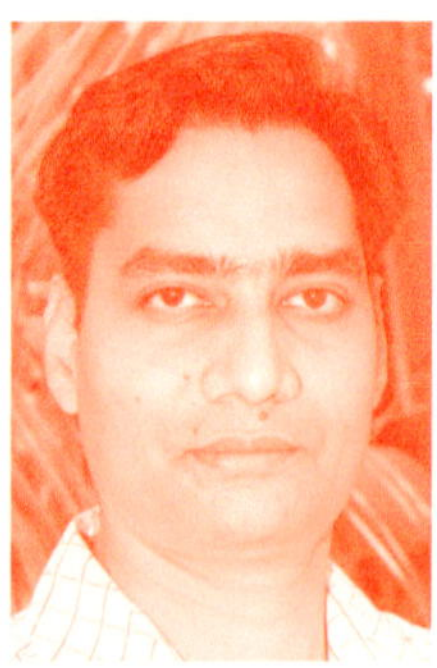
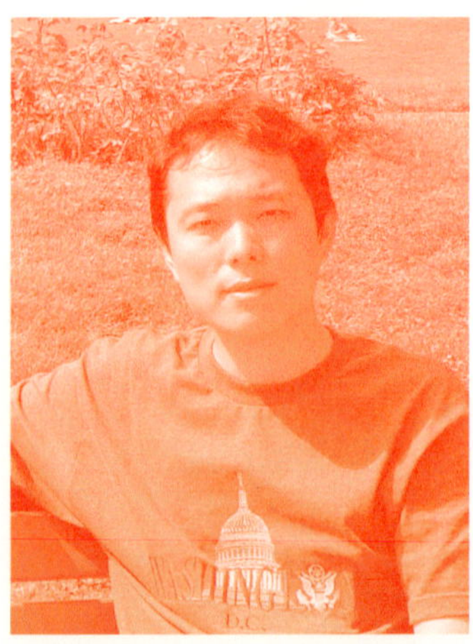
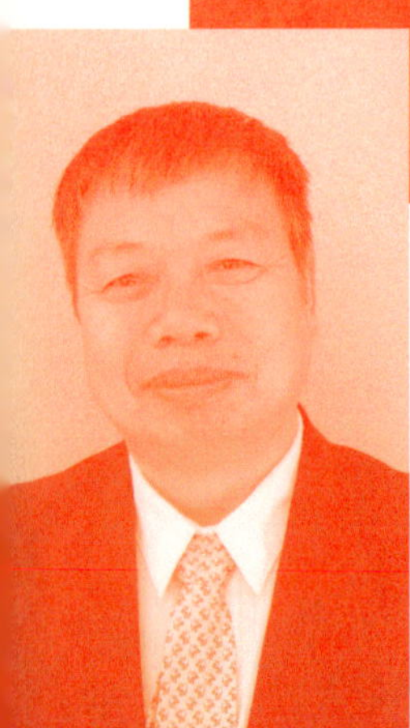
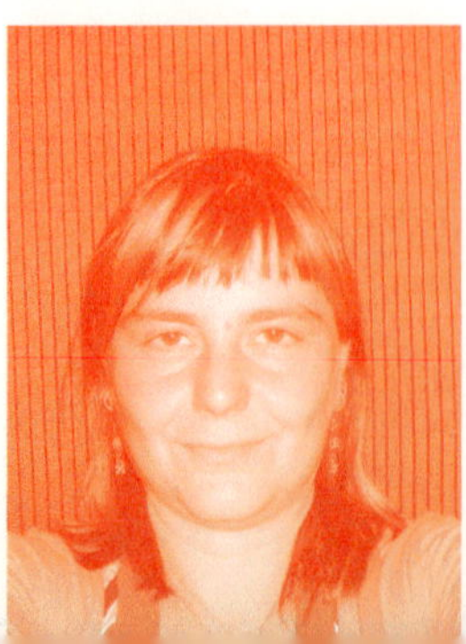

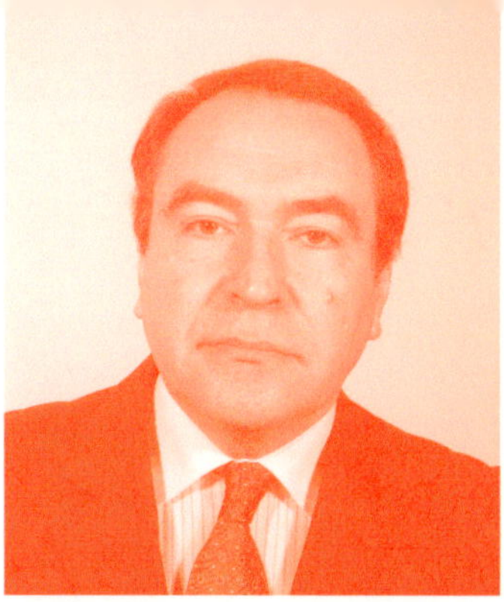
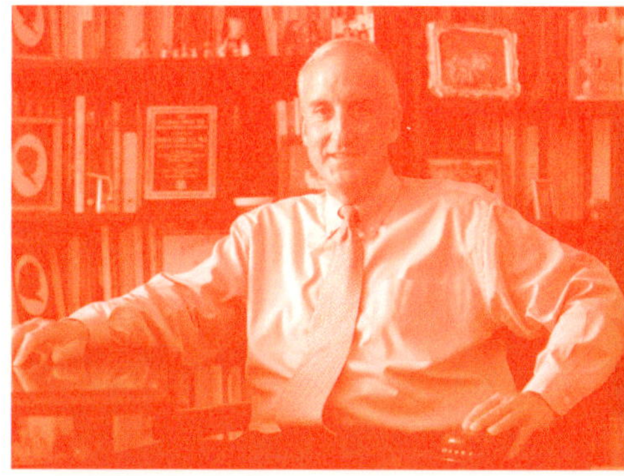
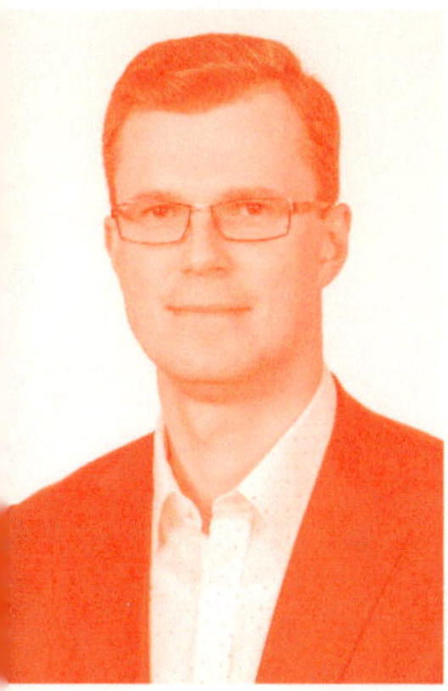
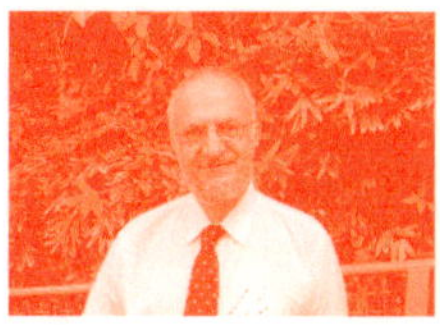
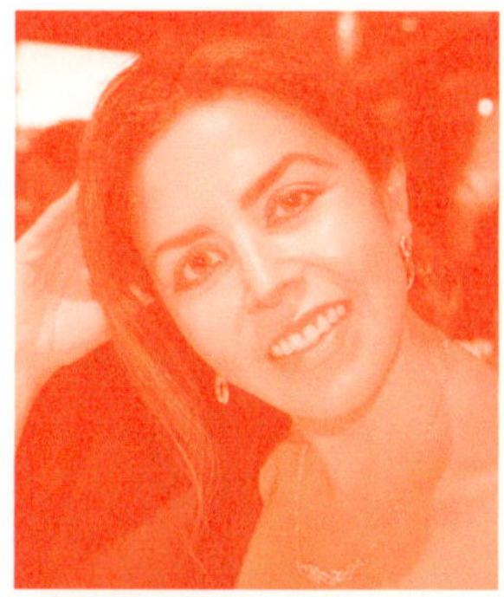

Supporting open minds since 2005

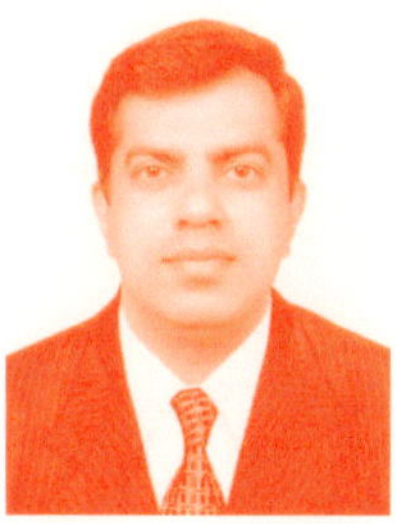
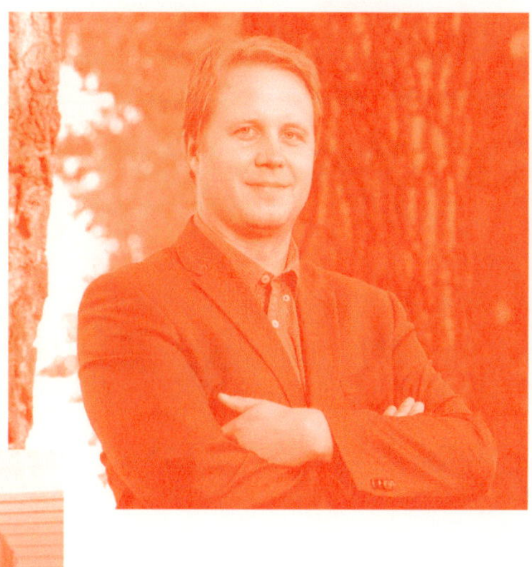
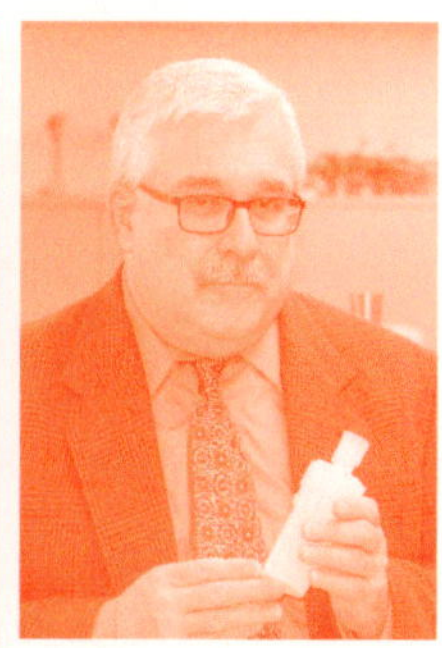
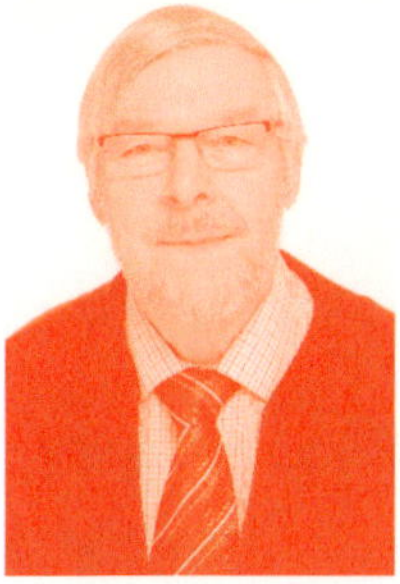
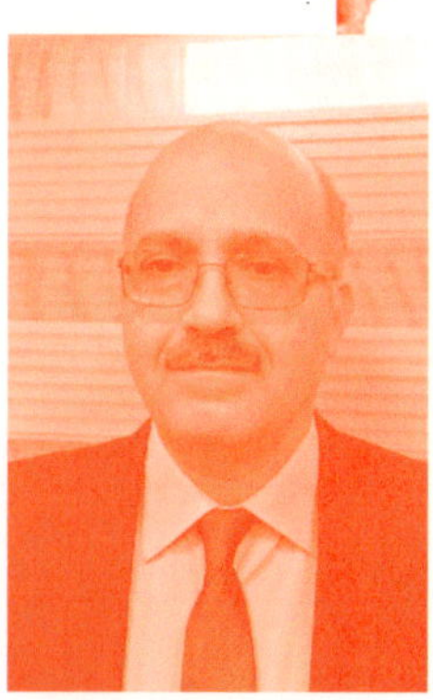
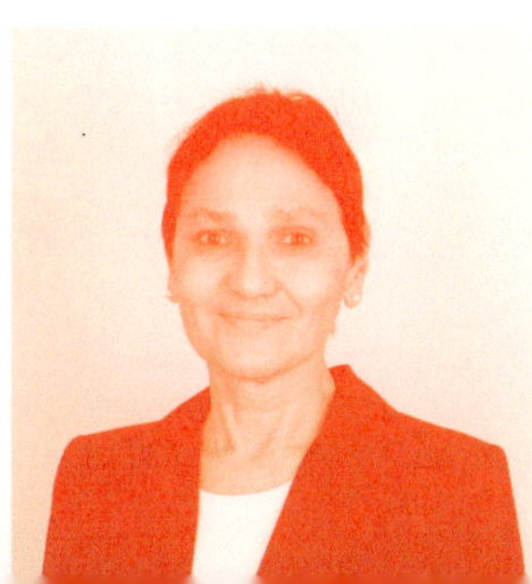
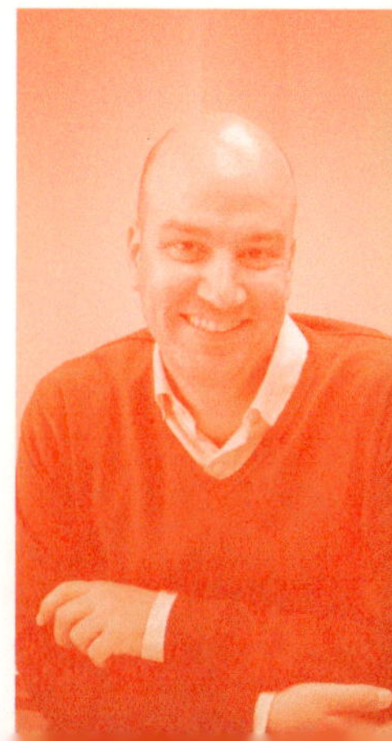

Novel Aspects on Motor Neuron Disease
http://dx.doi.org/10.5772/intechopen.73840
Edited by Humberto Foyaca Sibat and Lourdes de Fátima Ibañez-Valdés

Contributors
Silvia Olivera-Bravo, Junling Wang, Wei Li, Amruta Paranjape, Hema Biju, Rohit Das, Alok Sharma, Nandini Gokulchandran, Hemangi Sane, Prerna Badhe, Radhika Pradhan, Humberto Foyaca Sibat, Lourdes de Fátima Ibañez-Valdés

First published in London, United Kingdom, 2020 by IntechOpen
IntechOpen is the global imprint of INTECHOPEN LIMITED, registered in England and Wales, registration number: 11086078, 7th floor, 10 Lower Thames Street, London, EC3R 6AF, United Kingdom
Printed in Croatia

British Library Cataloguing-in-Publication Data
A catalogue record for this book is available from the British Library

Additional hard and PDF copies can be obtained from orders@intechopen.com

Novel Aspects on Motor Neuron Disease
Edited by Humberto Foyaca Sibat and Lourdes de Fátima Ibañez-Valdés
p. cm.
Print ISBN 978-1-83880-773-3
Online ISBN 978-1-83880-774-0
eBook (PDF) ISBN 978-1-83880-800-6

For EU product safety concerns:
IN TECH d.o.o., Prolaz Marije Krucifikse Kozulić 3, 51000 Rijeka, Croatia, info@intechopen.com or visit our website at intechopen.com.

Meet the editors

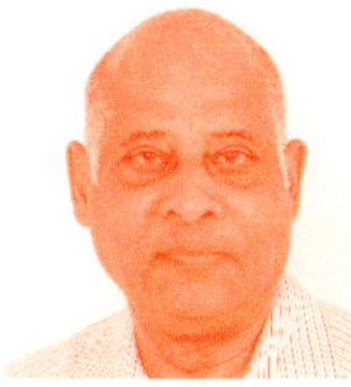

Humberto Foyaca Sibat, born on May 3, 1948 in Havana City, Cuba, graduated as a Medical Doctor from Havana University in 1971. He has been a first degree specialist in neurology since 1975 and Second Degree Specialist of Neurology since 1984. He has also achieved his PhD, MSc, Full Professor and Full Scientist Researcher. Dr. Foyaca is working as an Associate Professor in the Faculty of Health Sciences at Walter Sisulu University (South Africa) and Nelson Mandela Central Hospital in Mthatha as a Head of Department of Neurology since 1997. Dr. Foyaca is a member of 15 medical societies. He has presented more than 360 papers in national and international medical conferences. He has been invited to deliver key lectures several times. He has edited six books, and published more than 70 papers in peer-reviewed medical journals. Since 1992, he has been the Editor-in-Chief of the Internet Journal of Neurology.

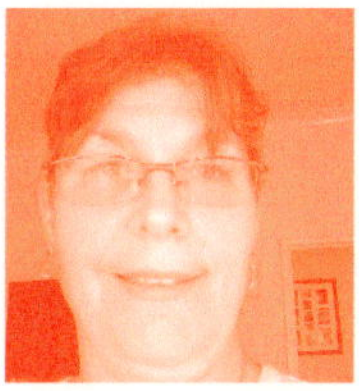

Dr. Lourdes de Fátima Ibañez-Valdés was born on October 13, 1963 in Havana City, Cuba. She graduated as a Medical Doctor from Havana University in 1998. She is also a specialist in family medicine, has her MSc in neuro-infectology, and is an aggregated scientist researcher at the Cuban Academy of Sciences. Currently she works for Department of Neurology at Walter Sisulu University, Nelson Mandela Academic Central Hospital in Mthatha, Eastern Cape Province, South Africa where she is the Head of Epilepsy and NCC-clinic. She has presented more than 60 papers at national and international medical conferences, published 8 chapters in text books and more than 40 articles in peer-reviewed journals. She is a member of 10 medical societies worldwide.

Contents

Preface

Motor Neuron Disease (MND) continues to be a progressive loss of structure and function of neurons in the cerebral cortex, brainstem, and the spinal cord. Usually the loss of specific functions precedes the death of affected neurons, and the related clinical features depend on localization and degree of neurodegeneration. Amyotrophic Lateral Sclerosis (ALS) is the more common clinical presentation and MND is also related to mitochondrial dysfunctions, increased oxidative stress and atypical protein assemblies. MND continues to be a serious health problem leading to death in few years' times in most of the patients. Before death, patients suffer from weakness or paralysis, muscle wasting and fasciculation, dysphagia, dysarthria and several complications. There are two forms of this fatal disease: sporadic, with no known genetic component, and familial, which makes up about 5% of all ALS cases. Among the familial cases, approximately 20% are caused by dominantly inherited mutations in the Cu/Zn superoxide dismutase (SOD1) gene, with more than 100 known mutations.

This is the second book that we have edited on ALS/MND. To edit this book, we have provided the best, safest, most confident and novel science information to our readers after following a rigorous process. All chapters were screened and analysed by a strict peer-review process, followed by corrections made by authors and the Academic Editor. Then a second revision was made by authors and editors performed the final review. It is important to highlight that after the peer-review process, all chapters were reviewed twice or even more to be accepted for publication. The chapter written by the Editor was also screened by another peer-review team.

In this book, the readers will find a compilation of state-of-the-art reviews about aetiology, therapies, investigations, the molecular basis of disease progression and clinical manifestations, and the genetics familial ALS, as well as novel diagnostic criteria.

An update aspect on ALS sourced 5 chapters from some of the world's top central nervous system researchers and neurologists to provide a timely review of the latest developments in MND/ALS, covering experimental animal models, genetics, clinical aspects and treatment options, amongst others.

Contributors from different countries have collaborated enthusiastically and efficiently to create this reader-friendly and comprehensive work covering the topics with many explanatory figures, tables and photos to enhance legibility and make the book clinically useful. Countless hours have gone into writing these chapters, precious free time to be dedicated to our family, relatives and friends have been sacrificed but at the end, we all are very proud of this book.

Every effort has been made to check the novel information given in this book but it is important for our readers to scrutinize other information arriving considering it is a dynamic process for learning. We all attempted to include valuable updated information for all issues mentioned in this book. Every effort has been made in the preparation and editing of this book to ensure that the information given is correct, but it is possible that errors have been overlooked. Finally, we would like to highlight that we reviewed all controversial matters and our medical criteria and scientist's opinions have been expressed with modesty, honesty and respect but the reader is advised to refer to other published information from other editorial houses and other reference works to check accuracy.

First of all, we would like to thank IntechOpen, who unconditionally supported us in editing this book. Special thanks should be given to my Author Service Managers, Ms. Dragana Manestar and Natalia Reinic, Ana Pantar, Andrea Koric and Romina Skomersic. They gave me support and encouragement to complete my previous editorial jobs successfully. For this book I had the supervision of Ms Dolores Kuzelj as Author Service Manager.

Currently, some of my previous chapters have reached more than 2000 downloads!

Our family have graciously tolerated the precious time spent on this project.

Fortunately, Mom, Dad and my first daughter Zayra Susana from heaven continue to inspire me. My second daughter, Lorna Maria (36 years old), and Fatima Susana Adolfina (10 years old) encouraged me to continue moving forward with persistence. My son Thabo Humberto Jorge (11 years old) both asked me to play games and to go for bike riding and these helped me to relax and to find new ideas but unfortunately I could not stay with them all times. My wife and the rest of my family contributed to this project and my wife was also my main collaborator - all of them deserve my deep gratitude.

Another token of gratitude must be delivered to all authors and collaborators for their patience and tolerance of the lost evenings, nights, weekends, holidays and free time spent on this project.

Special thanks go to Walter Sisulu University (WSU). Many thanks to Prof. Wilson Akpan: Director of Research & Development of WSU, Prof. AJ Mbokazi: Dean of the Faculty of Health Sciences (WSU), Prof. Thozama Dubula: Head of Department of General Medicine and Therapeutic, Dr. Mdledle and Dr. Nodikida: Acting Governor General: Clinical Governance of Nelson Mandela Central Hospital and Mrs. NP Makwedeni: Chief Executive Officer of Nelson Mandela Central Hospital for their understanding and professional support.

In the end, I extend my deepest sense of appreciation to Dr. Jorge Delgado Bustillo: Head of the National Unit for International Cooperation in Health, for the unconditional support received.

Humberto Foyaca Sibat
Professor,
Head of Department of Neurology,
Faculty of Health Sciences,
Walter Sisulu University,
Mthatha, South Africa

Dr. Lourdes de Fátima Ibañez-Valdés
Department of Neurology,
Nelson Mandela Academic Central Hospital,
Faculty of Health Sciences,
Walter Sisulu University,
Mthatha, South Africa

Section 1

Last Update on Motor Neuron Disease

Chapter 1

Introductory Chapter: Introduction to Novel Aspects on Motor Neuron Disease

Humberto Foyaca Sibat and Lourdes de Fátima Ibañez Valdés

1. Introduction

Motor neuron disease (MND) represents a wide and heterogeneous expanding group of diseases affecting the upper or lower motor neurons, mainly represented by amyotrophic lateral sclerosis (ALS), primary lateral sclerosis (PLS), progressive muscular atrophy (PMA), and progressive bulbar palsy. ALS is a disease of motor neuron degeneration in the cerebral hemisphere, brainstem, and spinal cord with a fatal prognosis in most of the cases due to a progressive paralysis of the diaphragm and other respiratory muscles leading to respiratory dysfunction and failure. Another recently recognized hallmark of ALS pathogenesis is vascular pathology apart from central nervous system capillary injury and microvascular impairment outside of the CNS [1].

2. Comments

Our first chapter is about stem cell therapy as a novel and promising modality for the treatment of ALS/MND. Robust safety profiles, low risk to benefit ratio, and ease of access make this approach a strong contender in the race against ALS/MND. Our authors concluded that this procedure is not a curative treatment, but a combinatorial approach integrating stem cell therapy, intensive neurorehabilitation, and current pharmacotherapeutic agents (e.g., Riluzole, Lithium, etc.) may be the best way forward. This chapter was written early last year (2019), but unfortunately, a prolonged editorial process impeded to publish this information at due time. However, we reviewed the medical literature and found that the abovementioned information has been confirmed recently (March 2020) by other authors [2].

In this book, we discussed about the pathogenic contribution of a subtype of aberrant glial phenotype into the progression and output of the neurodegenerative disease ALS and concluded that aberrant astrocytes or more generally aberrant glial cells are among the most important players in CNS damage causing deleterious effects through many potential pathological mechanisms, mostly sustained on their exacerbated proliferation together with their unprecedented neurotoxicity suggest that controlling these populations seems at least equally important than maintenance or restoration of homeostatic astrocyte functions to achieve CNS protection and repair. Another authors also suggest that aberrant glial cells (AbGC) isolated from the spinal cords of adult paralytic SOD1G93A rats exhibit highly proliferative and neurotoxic properties and may contribute to disease progression [4]. Same authors also established that mitochondrial dysfunction and neurotoxicity that can

IntechOpen

be reduced by dichloroacetate (DCA), a metabolic modulator that has been used in humans, show beneficial effects on disease outcome in SOD1G93A mice. They also highlight that DCA treatment of AbGC reduced extracellular lactate levels indicating that the main recognized DCA action targets the pyruvate dehydrogenase kinase/pyruvate dehydrogenase complex, and the results confirmed that AbGC metabolic phenotype is related to their toxicity to MNs and indicated that its modulation can reduce glial mediated pathology in the spinal cord [3]. At this point, it is important to emphasize that neuronal cell death is the main pathological feature of chronic neurodegenerative diseases (NDs) like ALS. A common hallmark of several NDs is the accumulation and aggregation of proteins; such proteins are thought to be primarily turned over by autophagy. Therefore, autophagy is considered a critical ND-protective pathway, which opens up potential new therapeutic interventions, and some authors have been considering the roles of autophagy and its contribution to neurodegeneration in neurons and concluded that little is known about the functions and disease contribution of the autophagy machinery in glia cells [4].

The next chapter of this book is related to the structural and functional consequences of the SMA-linked missense mutations of the survival motor neuron protein, where the authors deliver a brief update of the structural and functional consequences of the missense mutations of this SMA protein. There is another before published chapter where the same author investigates how SMA-linked mutations of SMN1 lead to structural/functional deficiency of SMN, and a set of computational analysis of SMN-related structures was conducted, described, and highlighted three residues of SMN (Asp44, Glu134, and Gln136), and the electrostatic basis of how the SMA-linked missense mutations of the three residues cause structural/functional deficiency of SMN and also a possibility of SMN's Lys45 and Asp36 acting as two electrostatically stabilizing clips at the SMN-Gemin2 complex structure interface [5].

Mutations to the gene encoding superoxide dismutase-1 (SOD1) were the first genetic elements discovered that cause motor neuron disease (MND). Around 10 years back, the unique way to test ALS-related gene was SOD1 sequencing. Based on this postulate, we approved to include into this project a novel review about the current understanding of ALS-related genes, summarize the worldwide ALS distribution feature by frequency of occurrence in different regions, and outline the genetic testing consideration, within many advances in the field of ALS genetics. In this chapter, the author highlights the recent advances in ALS gene map, genome-wide association study on ALS, genetic testing, and gene therapy.

Finally, we made a bibliography research about MND and the most recent advances on treatment and reviewed the most relevant papers published on the first trimester of 2019, but as was before-mentioned, this chapter is going to be published more than 1 year later when some of our information is already old-fashioned. Last year, we reviewed on novel information about edaravone, riluzole (already approved by Food and Drug Administration), nusinersen, EH301, 5Fluoroucil, Tryptophan, RNS60, Rasagiline, Tirasemtiv, Aquaporin, Fasudil, and Lunasil. In order to deliver to our reader community, more novel information about MND/ALS is important to highlight other procedure that has been proposed for treatment such as the multifaceted role of kinases in ALS. The comprehensive regulation of kinases, however, a better understanding of the disturbances in the kinome network in ALS, is needed to properly target specific kinases in the clinic. Different kinases have been recently involved in TDP-43 phosphorylation. Among these, protein casein kinase-1 is the first kinase identified to phosphorylate TDP-43 *in vivo*, followed by tau tubulin kinase 1 and cell division cycle kinase 7. Currently, it is recognized that TDP-43 proteinopathy characterized by truncation, ubiquitination, hyperphosphorylation, and/or nuclear depletion in neurons is the prominent and common pathological feature of sporadic and familiar ALS [6]. Some authors explored the effects of a chronic treatment with the compound IGS-2.7 in the TDP-43 (A315T) transgenic mouse model and found a significant decrease in the levels of phosphorylation of TDP-43 in sporadic ALS lymphoblast, while no differences were observed in control group, and they arrived to the following conclusion: prolonged treatment with IGS-2.7 prevents the phosphorylation of TDP-43 *in vivo* in the cord of TDP-43 transgenic mice, being this effect associated with an attenuation of most of the events that reflect the worsening of the pathological phenotype, then the inhibition of CK-1δ with the benzothiazole derivative IGS-2.7 may modulate TDP-43 toxicity *in vivo* by limiting TDP-43 phosphorylation, which could explain the benefits obtained with this drug candidate in the preservation of spinal motor neurons. Therefore, benzothiazole IGS-2.7 has neuroprotective properties and not only decreases TDP-43 phosphorylation in cells derived from ALS patients but also corrects the subcellular localization of TDP-43, preventing the abnormal cytosolic TDP-43 accumulation in ALS lymphoblasts [6].

For another hand, other authors reported that 185 miRNAs in serum of affected patients and controls confirmed a downregulation of miR-335-5p in ALS patients [7].

Because we are under obligation to deliver the most recent information about MND/ALS therapy to our reader's community, then we would like to comment about clinically used ebselen and related analogues to promote thermal stability of A4V SOD1 when binding to Cys111 only [8]. Ebselen is an organoselenium compound with activity similar to glutathione peroxidase [9]. Several studies have demonstrated the neuroprotective activity of ebselen, possibly via its anti-oxidant properties [10, 11]. The capacity of ebselen to decrease mitochondrial cellular toxicity caused by mutant SOD1 confirmed that this compound plays an important role in alleviating familial ALS [12].

Acknowledgements

We thank all authors and their relatives for the support received during the development of this project.

Author details

Humberto Foyaca Sibat* and Lourdes de Fátima Ibañez Valdés
Department of Neurology, Nelson Mandela Academic Central Hospital, Walter Sisulu University, Mthatha, South Africa

*Address all correspondence to: humbertofoyacasibat@gmail.com

References

[1] Foyaca HS, Ibanez-Valdes L de F. Introduction to update in amyotrophic lateral sclerosis and review of this condition in sportsmen. Chapter I. In: Foyaca HS, Ibanez Valdes L, editors. Update on Amyotrophic Lateral Sclerosis. Rijeka: IntechOpen; 2016. DOI: 10.5772/64608. Available from: http://www.intechopen.com/myprofile/index/dashboard. ISBN: 978-953-51-2601-0

[2] Garbuzova-Davis S, Shell R, Mustafa H, Hailu S, Willing AE, Sanberg PR, et al. Advancing stem cell therapy for repair of damaged lung microvasculature in amyotrophic lateral sclerosis. Cell Transplantation. 2020;**29**:963689720913494. DOI: 10.1177/0963689720913494

[3] Martínez-Palma L, Miquel E, Lagos-Rodríguez V, Barbeito L, Cassina A, Cassina P. Mitochondrial modulation by dichloroacetate reduces toxicity of aberrant glial cells and gliosis in the SOD1G93A rat model of amyotrophic lateral sclerosis. Neurotherapeutics. 2019;**16**(1):203-215

[4] Strohm L, Behrends C. Glia-specific autophagy dysfunction in ALS. Seminars in Cell & Developmental Biology. 2020;**99**:172-182

[5] Li W. How do SMA-linked mutations of SMN1 lead to structural/functional deficiency of the SMA protein? PLOS One. 2017;**12**(6):-e0178519

[6] Martínez-González L, Rodríguez-Cueto C, Cabezudo D, Bartolomé F, Andrés-Benito P, et al. Motor neuron preservation and decrease of *in vivo* TDP-43 phosphorylation by protein CK-1δ kinase inhibitor treatment. Scientific Reports. 2020;**10**:4449. DOI: 10.1038/s41598-020-61265-y

[7] De Luna N, Turon-Sans J, Cortes-Vicente E, Carrasco-Rozas A, et al. Downregulation of miR-335-5P in amyotrophic lateral sclerosis can contribute to neuronal mitochondrial dysfunction and apoptosis. Scientific Reports. 2020;**10**:4308. DOI: 10.1038/s41598-020-61246-1

[8] Chantadul V, Wright GSA, Amporndanai K, Shahid M, Antonyuk SV, Washbourn G, et al. Ebselen as template for stabilization of A4V mutant dimer for motor neuron disease therapy. Communications Biology. 2020;**3**:97. DOI: 10.1038/s42003-020-0826-3

[9] Takasago T, Peters EE, Graham DI, Masayasu H, Macrae IM. Neuroprotective efficacy of ebselen, an anti-oxidant with anti-inflammatory actions, in a rodent model of permanent middle cerebral artery occlusion. British Journal of Pharmacology. 1997;**122**:1251-1256. DOI: 10.1038/sj.bjp.0701426

[10] Kalayci M et al. Neuroprotective effects of ebselen on experimental spinal cord injury in rats. Neurochemical Research. 2005;**30**:403-410. DOI: 10.1007/s11064-005-2615-2

[11] Martini F et al. A multifunctional compound ebselen reverses memory impairment, apoptosis and oxidative stress in a mouse model of sporadic Alzheimer's disease. Journal of Psychiatric Research. 2019;**109**:107-117. DOI: 10.1016/j.jpsychires.2018.11.021

[12] Wood-Allum CA et al. Impairment of mitochondrial anti-oxidant defence in SOD1-related motor neuron injury and amelioration by ebselen. Brain. 2006;**129**:1693-1709. DOI: 10.1093/brain/awl118

Chapter 2

Contribution of Aberrant Astrocytes to Motor Neuron Damage and Death in the SOD1G93A Rat Experimental Model of ALS

Gabriel Otero Damianovich, Olga Cristina Parada, Pablo Díaz-Amarilla, Eugenia Eloísa Isasi, Carmen Isabel Bolatto Pereira and Silvia Olivera-Bravo

Abstract

Amyotrophic lateral sclerosis (ALS) is an incurable paralyzing disease characterized by motor neuron death and glial reactivity. Superoxide dismutase 1 (SOD1) are among the most frequent alterations found in around 15–20% of ALS inheritable forms. Mutant SOD1 murine models mimic main human ALS features and allow purposing that pathological mechanisms include defective communication between neural cells together with astrocyte preponderant roles in disease progression. Years ago, a subset of the most neurotoxic aberrant astrocytes (AbAs) was obtained from spinal cords of SOD1G93A rats. AbA cultures show an exponential growing yield since the early symptoms of the disease up to the terminal stages. In cultures, AbAs present unprecedented toxicity to motor neurons, increased proliferation, loss of mature astrocyte markers, as well as extreme ER stress and abundant extracellular matrix components. Strikingly, AbA phenotype seems to be changing along few passages suggesting its signaling and features may accompany disease progression. However, the link between main AbA features and their highest motor neuron toxicity is not yet completely understood. Here, we reviewed ALS underlying pathological mechanisms in association to AbA phenotype, to collaborate with identification of the most relevant processes that seem crucially involved in the triggering or maintenance of neurotoxicity.

Keywords: aberrant astrocytes, motor neuron death, non-cell autonomous disease

1. Introduction

This chapter will discuss the pathogenic contribution of a subtype of aberrant glial phenotype into the progression and output of the neurodegenerative disease amyotrophic lateral sclerosis (ALS). Complete understanding of neuronal and glial cells roles and communication is necessary to unravel disease processes and mechanisms. This will further allow the improvement of more focused therapeutic interventions aimed at reducing disease severity and positively impact on diagnosis, therapeutic management, and patients' care.

2. ALS

ALS is an adult onset neurodegenerative disease characterized by progressive loss of spinal, brain stem, and cortical motor neurons, leading to fatal paralysis within 1–5 years since the onset of symptoms that include tremor, muscle weakness, and spasticity [1–3]. ALS affects up to 2:100,000 persons per year; has a life risk around 1:500–1:1000; and exhibits a little predominance of men over women affected [4]. Although ALS is a sporadic multifactorial disease resulting from yet unknown interactions among environment, genes, and epigenetic modifications, genetics seemed to be the predominant factor for the risk of developing the disease [5], and more than 10% of ALS patients are linked to inheritable genetic abnormalities. Dominant mutations in the mitochondrial enzyme Cu/Zn superoxide dismutase-1 (SOD1) seem responsible for up to 1% of the total ALS cases and about 20% of the familial types [4, 6, 7]. Missense mutations in the 43 kDa transactive response DNA/RNA-binding protein (TDP-43) [8] and in fused in sarcoma/translocated in liposarcoma (FUS/TLS) accounted each one for up to 5% of dominantly inherited familial ALS cases [9, 10]. Mutations in the open reading frame 72 on chromosome 9 (C9ORF72) that results in up to thousands of G4C2 hexanucleotide repeats in one allele are found in up to 40 and 7% of the ALS familial and sporadic cases, respectively [11]. There are other genes involved in ALS familial subtypes, but its contribution to the disease is significantly lower in terms of the affected individual number. Regarding to the pathological pathways linking genetic abnormalities to ALS, SOD1 mutations seem to be related to neuronal damage because of abnormal protein folding causes unstable conformations, intracellular inclusion bodies or toxic oligomers, as well as pathological interactions with several proteins [3]. TDP-43 and FUS/TLS mutations are linked to altered RNA processing, transport, and quality control; whereas, G4C2 repeats might sequestrate RNA-binding proteins impairing the regulation of the RNA targets [12, 13] or causing epigenetic changes that decreased C9ORF72 expression [14, 15]. However, up to now, it is not completely understood how single mutations in one protein could elicit the ALS pathological cascades and how these cascades may finally cause a common neuropathological hallmark that is characterized by aggregation and accumulation of neuronal proteinaceous inclusions that in addition, are found in other neurodegenerative conditions including Alzheimer disease.

2.1 Animal models and non-cell autonomous mechanisms in ALS

To understand the different pathological mechanisms involved in ALS, many experimental models from yeast to rodents have been developed. Whereas, models in lower animals are powerful genetic tools and offer advantages related to short life span and easy handling, distance with mammal nervous systems constitute major limitations when studying human neurodegeneration [16, 17]. Mice and rats are closer to human brain anatomy and complexity, but are not good genetic tools and their lifespan makes necessary the over-expression of mutant human proteins several-fold times to mimic the disease [4], causing the risk that the number of copies over-expressed influence the model by itself. In spite of this, animal models appear as the best approaches to study ALS patho-mechanisms, at least until the employment of inducible pluripotent cells obtained from human patients becomes a well-known and controlled technology.

The first successful ALS models, yet under current extensive use, were developed over-expressing different single mutations of human SOD1 (SOD1G93A, SOD1G37R, and SOD1G85R) in mice or rats [18–20]. Most of the models that overexpress SOD1 present an age-dependent progressive motor syndrome that mimics some pathological features of the human disease [4, 20]. In addition, it seems that pathological features elicited do not derive from the loss of SOD1 catalytic activity but from a yet unknown gain-of-function [4, 20]. Among the highest contributions of murine SOD1 models to the ALS knowledge is the introduction of the non-cell autonomous mechanism concept in which the exclusive neuronal presence of mutant SOD1 did not cause motor neuron death. This implies that motor neuron disease results from the involvement of at least two different cell types. Therefore, a defective cell-cell communication between motor neurons and surrounding glial cells seems actively participating in motor neuron death through not completely understood mechanisms. Pioneer works made in LoxSOD1G37R/GFAP-Cre^{+} mice [21] or specifically excising the mutant SOD1 transgene from different glial cell types in mice [22, 23] showed that astrocytes [21] and microglial cells [22] play active roles in ALS progression. In support of the non-cell autonomous mechanisms in SOD1 models, reactive astrocytes obtained from transgenic rats or mice [24–26], and from patients of sporadic and familial motor neuron diseases [27, 28] caused neurotoxicity to motor neurons even in cases in which SOD1 is not involved [28].

Other ALS models in rodents were not as clear as those over-expressing mutated SOD1. Transgenic animals expressing mutations of TDP-43-, FUS/TLS-, or C9ORF72-linked ALS produced controversial results without a clear association between each mutation and motor neuron disease, in spite of having motor neuron damage, proteinaceous inclusions, and astrogliosis [29, 30]. Despite these drawbacks, ALS models valuably contribute to make the concept that disruption at systemic, cellular, and molecular levels likely result in many different interacting mechanisms and multiple factors, and that a particular combination of factors and mechanisms likely determine the singularity of each case thus explains the heterogeneity of the human disease.

3. Contribution of aberrant glial phenotypes to ALS pathogenesis

SOD1 models support the concept of ALS as a non-cell autonomous disease in which the reactive astrocyte phenotypes that are produced in the injuring environment greatly contribute to motor neuron death. Astrocytes are the most abundant glial cells in the mammal brain and those responsible for the maintenance of CNS homeostasis [31–34]. During injury, CNS homeostasis is lost and astrocytes respond in a process usually called astrogliosis, in which cells became reactive, highly proliferative and with morphological and functional changes that usually result in decreased protection together with activation of injuring cascades to neurons and oligodendrocytes, further affecting the whole CNS [31–37]. Depending on the injury type and context, astrocyte response can become chronic causing a long lasting state characterized by glial scar, structural tissue rearrangement and impeded repair, as well as a permanent imbalance among homeostatic supportive and gain of neurotoxic functions, all potentially participating in the triggering and progression of several neurological diseases [3, 31–35, 37, 38]. Remarkably, astrocytes also contribute to maintain astrogliosis through autocrine and paracrine signaling [35, 38, 39], thus causing a positive feedback that widespread reactivity and dependent injuring cascades perpetuating CNS damage.

A striking question that remained unanswered until recently was to know if all of the astrocytes that share the same injuring environment respond in the same way or if some of them adopt the worse aberrant phenotypes that account for most of the neurotoxic effects. Trying to unravel this question, when we were studying spinal cord astrocyte phenotypes along the symptomatic phase of the rat SOD1G93A ALS experimental model, we isolated a novel type of aberrant astrocyte-like cells (AbAs) from the spinal cord of paralytic animals whose number exponentially increased toward the terminal stages of the disease [40]. AbAs proliferated faster than astrocytes from neonates or adult wild-type rats and were exceptionally toxic to embryonic motor neurons grown in culture, suggesting a link between their emergence and progression of the paralysis that is a characteristic in the SOD1G93A ALS rat model. Moreover, AbAs did not express distinctive markers that clearly allow distinguishing from typical astrocytes; but present peculiar functional and ultrastructural features that suggest a distinctive phenotype. Among the most remarkable features that AbAs possess, Jiménez-Riani et al. [41] describe their permanent absence of contact inhibition that allowed them to grow in multiple layers and arrange in 3D-cell aggregates that adopt a helicoidal pattern with a central core of extracellular matrix surrounded by cells. In addition, AbAs cytoskeleton does not have intermediate filaments but a significant abundance of microtubules and mitochondria, and ER stress have a restricted perinuclear location suggesting disturbed organelle trafficking that may be associated to alteration in microtubule network or Golgi fragmentation [42]. Furthermore, mitochondria from AbAs are small, electron dense matrix and with few crests; all, comparable to what was described early in models and human ALS [43, 44]. AbAs also have prominent ER with extremely swollen cisternae, some of them degenerating, and express high levels of some ER stress markers [45–47], as well as abundant lipid droplets close to ER and to mitochondria. Their cytoplasm is enriched in diverse vesicles with abundant signs of secretion including extracellular vesicles that can be distinguished by MET and SEM in cultures as well as expression of protein that marks secretion granules [41, 48, 49]. AbAs are also highly positive to the autophagy marker LC3B [50] and present cells' autophagic vesicles and residual bodies [51, 52], likely showing signs of increased autophagy that may allow cells coping with ER stress by favoring the clearance of misfolded proteins [53].

Recently, we confirmed that AbAs were not isolated from the cervical spinal cord of paralytic animals. Instead, the cultures obtained from the cervical spinal cord were similar to the age-matched wild type non-transgenic rats, sharing a low rate of proliferation and resembling a phagocytic microglia morphology that persists throughout the cell culture. Similarities also include low survival along few passages together with absence of complete phenotypic transition to flat cells like astrocytes (**Figure 1**). Therefore, AbAs might result as a local lumbar response to damage, acting similar to astrocytes when react stereotypically depending on injury type, location, and signaling [32].

In addition, we have found that some AbAs critical features are changing during few passages, as occurring with their most prominent markers S100β and glial glutamate transporter GLT1. Meanwhile, there were no evident morphological differences between low (LP) (~4–7) and high passages (HP) (~14–18) (**Figure 2A**), since cultured AbAs proliferated without replicative senescence, S100β expression levels decreased ≅98% (**Figure 2B**), suggesting that this aberrant phenotype may exhibit some plasticity along time. S100β is a well-known danger-associated molecular pattern (DAMP) which downstream trigger the transcription of nuclear factor NFKB that further may elicit increased expression and release of pro-inflammatory cytokines [54, 55]. Given that S100β appears to integrate AbAs

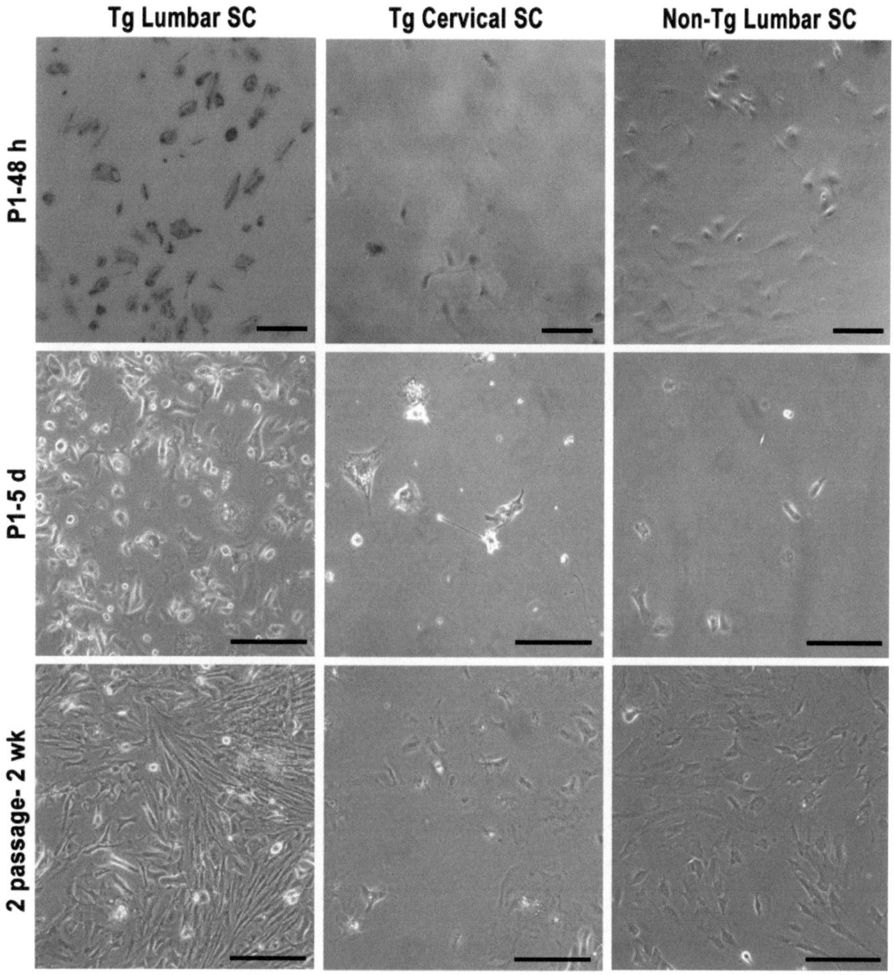

Figure 1.
Morphological appearance of AbAs throughout the cell culture. Light microscopy examination of cells isolated from symptomatic cervical and lumbar spinal cord of transgenic (Tg cervical SC and Tg lumbar SC) or age-matched non-transgenic animals (No Tg lumbar SC) at 48 h, 5 days and 2 weeks after dissection. Note that AbA cells are recovered only from the lumbar spinal cord of transgenic animals whereas the cultures obtained from the cervical spinal cord of the same animals have similar characteristics to the age-matched wild type non-transgenic rats. Adherent cell population is heterogenous with very bright cells that resemble microglial cells and others elongated similar to astrocytes. Scale bar = 150 μm (first line) and 100 μm (second and third lines).

cytoskeletal elements, we cannot discard that S100β downregulated expression may cause cytoskeleton instability, a characteristic that is linked to exacerbated proliferative capacity as found in AbAs [56]. Thus, decreasing S100β might constitute a reinforcing proliferation feedback that may underlie AbAs invasive properties as disease progressed. We have also found that GLT1 expression levels also decreased strongly along AbAs passages (≅94%, **Figure 2B**), worsening its poor expression which can also aggravated excitotoxic damage [31].

Concurrence of all of the features makes AbAs a unique aberrant phenotype with unprecedented neurotoxicity, which may rely in the yet unknown combination of ER stress, lipid droplet accumulation, abundant extracellular matrix, secretory granules, and exacerbated proliferation. Likely, all these events causing the active production of proteinaceous or lipidic soluble factors that act by itself or reinforce the defective cell-contact properties produced by loss of contact inhibition [41].

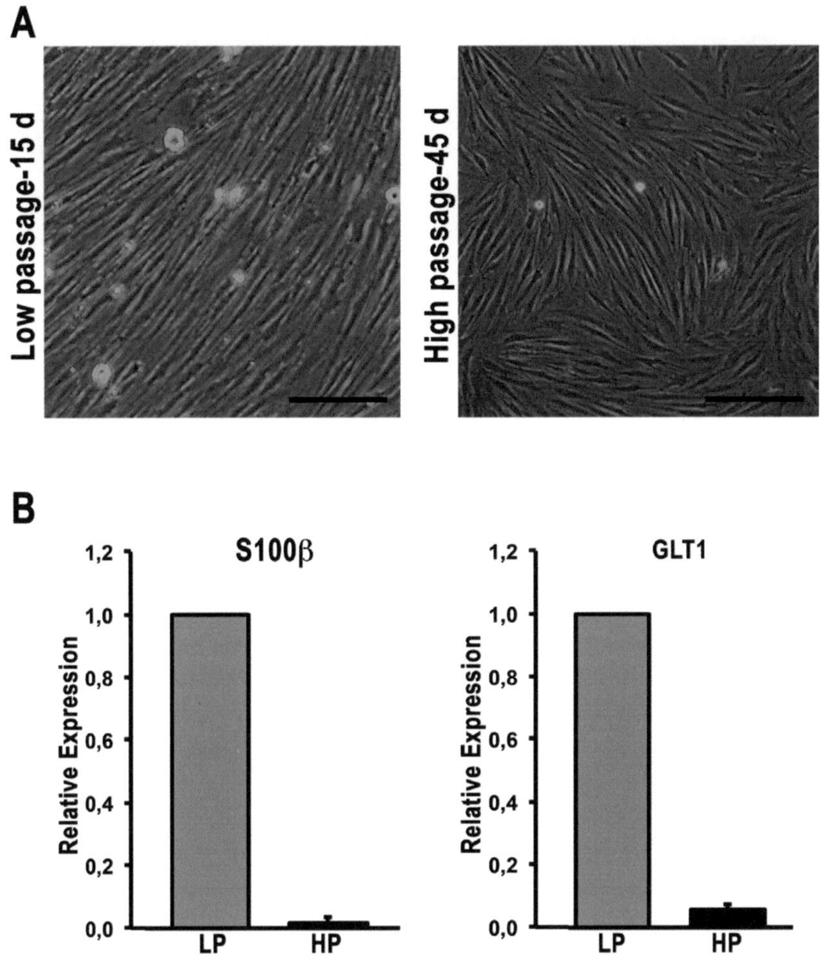

Figure 2.
Morphology and gene expression in AbAs at low and high cell passages. A. Representative light microscopy images of low (LP, left) and high (HP, right) passage cells from transgenic lumbar spinal cords showing their distinctive appearance of flatted elongated cells that appear very similar to astrocytes. Note the low number of bright microglial-like cells. Scale bar = 100 μm. B. Gene expression analysis in AbA cell cultures showing a down-regulation of S100β (left) and glutamate transporter GLT1 (right) in HP cells compared with LP cells (control). The expression levels for each gene were obtained by SYBR green qPCR and normalized to the actin transcripts. Data represent the mean ± the standard deviation for each group.

3.1 Mechanisms that might link AbA to ALS pathogenesis

The most important cellular processes implicated in ALS pathophysiology include ER stress and protein clearance, neuron-glia metabolic coupling, and energy homeostasis [57, 58]. Among their most remarkable features, AbAs exhibit a hardly coping extreme ER stress, as well as lipid droplets and disturbed mitochondrial morphology and trafficking [41]. ER stress is produced by the lack of balance between protein synthesis, folding, and degradation rates [59]. To recover ER homeostasis, cells activate the unfolded protein response (UPR) that orchestrates pro-adaptive and pro-death cellular responses that include protein synthesis decrease except for the effectors that mediates UPR [59–61]. ER stress's final outcome depends on stress duration, strength, and cell targets, and if not resolved, it becomes chronic and as one of the earliest perturbations in several neurodegenerative diseases [59]. Interestingly, ER stress is present in ALS experimental models, and is described as a predominant mechanism underlying motor neuron death in patients from sporadic and familial cases [46, 59, 62–66]. Furthermore, active UPR in AbAs may down regulate the expression of peptides and proteins that collaborate with neuron survival such as the most important cellular antioxidant defense glutathione or neurotrophins [3, 32]. Thus, although ER stress in AbAs did not cause their own death, it is highly probable that it affects neuron and oligodendrocyte survival in view of their high dependence on astrocyte support.

In close relationship with ER stress, AbAs are also much enriched in lipid droplets that appear near to mitochondria or ER cisternae [41]. Lipid droplets originate from the ER and are described as having a role in ER stress and clearance of protein aggregates as well as in energy homeostasis [67]. Protein turnover is critical for ALS because a number of mutations linked to ALS affect genes directly involved in protein clearance and homeostasis [58]. Lipid droplets appear associated with some of these proteins into the cytoplasm or the nucleus [67, 68], where they appear close and likely associated with the nuclear-naked organelles that control transcriptional activity, cell senescence, and protein degradation named as promyelocytic leukemia nuclear bodies [67, 69, 70], which in addition are found in cell nuclei of ALS patient brains co-localizing with ubiquitin and proteasome components in nuclear inclusions [71].

In brain, lipid droplets are found mainly in glial cells and help to provide fuel for neurons when energy is needed and glucose is scarce. At this time, lipid droplets turned over by cytoplasmic lipases and autophagy, providing fatty acid fuel for ATP production [67], thus playing a crucial role in the anaplerotic support [72]. However, overabundance of lipid droplets as seen in AbAs may suggest a disrupted lipid metabolism in which lipid droplets may not be digested thus decreasing the energy intermediate shuttle to neurons, which can influence motor neuron survival through limited anaplerosis. Lipidic dysfunction could also indirectly impact motor neuron survival as shown in mice over-expressing TDP-43, that beside displaying neurological symptoms and motor deficits, also present increased fat accumulation and adipocyte hypertrophy [73]. Conversely, TDP-43 depletion causes body fat reduction, increased fatty acid consumption, and rapid death [74], likely, because TDP-43 depletion blocks insulin-induced trafficking of glucose transporter Glut4 to the plasma membrane thus impairing glucose uptake and inducing a metabolic switch toward lipids for energy production. This has also been reported in SOD1 mouse models in which spinal cord neurons display decreased glucose usage [75], and a fat-rich diet restores body mass, delays disease onset, and extends life expectancy [57]. Moreover, excessive accumulation of lipid droplets in glial cells is a hallmark in many models of neurodegeneration, and it is usually linked to mitochondrial dysfunction and disease progression [72, 76, 77]. It also seemed enough to promote neurodegeneration by itself [76], therefore indicating that overabundance of lipid droplets in AbAs may have dual functions: for one side not only helping to the clearance of abnormal proteins, but also impairing anaplerotic support to neurons or even having direct neurotoxicity.

AbAs also show evidences of a high secretory activity, which also is described as being crucial to ALS neuronal damage. Although secretory granules seem a conserved protective response to conserve energy and allow recovery under stress conditions, sustained secretory activity of stress granules seems crucial to ALS pathogenesis [78]. Moreover, it has been demonstrated that chromogranins interact and co-localize with mutated misfolded SOD1 [79]; and can eventually act as chaperones to promote secretion of SOD1 mutants that once released may trigger microgliosis and neuronal death [79].

Absence of contact inhibition and exacerbated proliferation are other of the relevant features related to AbAs neurotoxic capacity. Contact inhibition that occurs when dividing normal cells contact adjacent ones is crucial to maintain tissue homeostasis [80, 81], thus constituting an important anticancer mechanism which lack unleashes cells to proliferate virtually unchecked. Although underlying mechanisms are mostly unknown, cell contact inhibition seems to occur when injury disrupts intercellular contacts achieving a proliferative status leading to an aggressive state associated with neoplasia [82] and malignant transformation [81]. Thus, AbAs, absence of contact inhibition seemed directly related to their exacerbated proliferation and invasive behavior during the final stages of the disease. In addition, abundance of EM components secreted by AbA cells may create a non-permissive microenvironment that potentiates invasive behavior apart from having a direct neurotoxic influence to motor neurons, as described in ALS astrocytes [83–85]. No one of each proposed mechanisms seem enough to explain AbAs unprecedented neurotoxicity. Instead, it likely results from the concurrence of many pathological pathways. However, it is also possible that one or two underlying mechanisms prevail over the rest and elicit most of AbAs deleterious effects. Identification of these prevalent mechanisms will be a valuable aid to design the best ALS treatment (**Table 1** and **Figure 3**).

(i) Absence of contact inhibition • Invasive phenotype [40, 41] • Lack of replicative senescence [40, 86] • Exacerbated proliferation [40, 86, 87]
(ii) Immature phenotype • Lack of gliofilaments [40, 41] • Defective differentiation [40, 41, 88]
(iii) Oxidative and ER stress • Mitochondrial dysfunction [89, 90] • Mitochondrial morphological alterations [41] • Defective oxidative phosphorylation [89, 90] • Dysfunction in energy homeostasis [24, 89, 91] • Dilated ER and degenerating ER cisternae [41] • Elevated expression of ER stress markers [41]
(iv) Altered lipid metabolism • Abundant lipid droplets close to mitochondria & ER [41] • Altered anaplerotic support [88]
(v) Intracellular inclusions • Intranuclear and intramitochondrial deposits [41] • Abundance of autophagic bodies [41]
(vi) Aberrant signaling • Extremely neurotoxic conditioned media [40] • Neurotoxic exosomes [90] • Abundance of secretory vesicles and secretory body markers [41]

Table 1.
A summary of AbAs potential pathogenic contribution to the main ALS hallmark. All of ALS main features are listened as (i)–(vi) together with each specific AbAs potential participation.

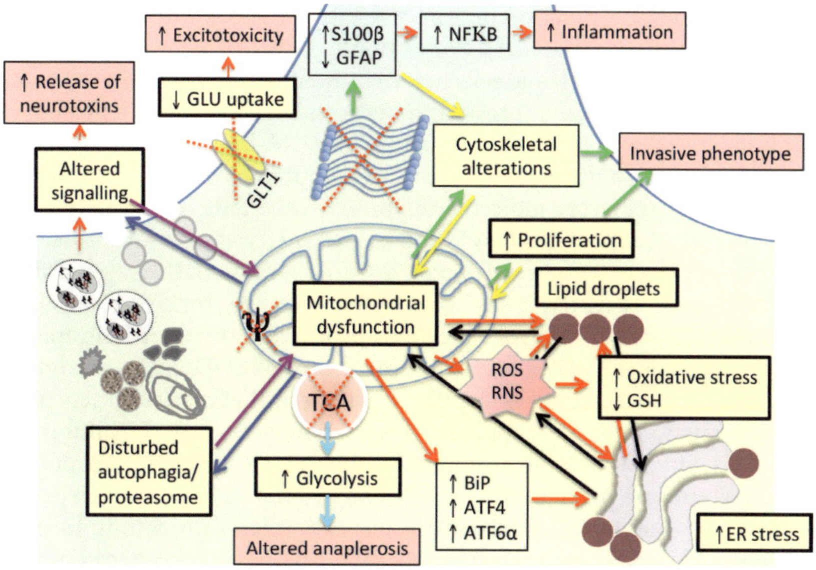

Figure 3.
AbAs: Cytotoxic effects and pathological events. AbAs present mitochondrial dysfunction associated to oxidative stress and ER stress as well as accumulation of lipid droplets, all causing a positive feedback that elicit and perpetuate cell damage (red and black arrows). Mitochondrial abnormalities together with cytoskeletal alterations are also involved in AbAs exacerbated proliferation and cytoskeleton instability both likely underlying the absence of contact inhibition and invasive phenotype as well as S100β-dependent inflammation cascades (green and yellow arrows). Progressive loss of the glutamate transporter GLT1 causes decreased glutamate uptake becoming neurons more expose to glutamate excitoxicity. Altered signaling and disturbed autophagia and proteasome functions caused the release of stress granules and soluble neurotoxins as well as the accumulation of cell detritus and inclusion bodies (violet and blue arrows). Finally, the lack of mitochondrial potential (represented as Ψ) caused increased glycolysis and deficient anaplerosis that alters the trophic and energetic support to neurons and oligodendrocytes (light blue).

4. ALS therapeutics focused on aberrant astrocytes

ALS is an old disease with a narrow offer of pharmacological approaches. Riluzole, an anti-glutamatergic drug, was the first compound authorized to be used in ALS, providing around of 3-month improvement in survival [92]. Recently, FDA approved the free radical scavenger edaravone, as the second compound to treat ALS, that seemed to have beneficial effects only on patients in an early stages of the disease that in addition satisfy a number of restricted criteria. In that population, edavarone showed a significantly smaller decline of Revised ALS Functional Rating Scale score compared with placebo [93]. A randomized phase III clinical trial that tested the effect of the tyrosine kinase inhibitor masitinib in ALS patients showed an improving in the functioning of ALS patients, and the combination with riluzole caused a delayed disease progression without adverse effects [94]. However, the narrow temporal windows that the two compounds approved offer obligates to search alternative avenues to treat the disease.

As astrocytes and microglial cells develop both protective and pathological functions its pharmacological targeting must be carefully evaluated. However, in view of the distinctive phenotype of AbAs, it seems rational to direct therapeutic treatments toward the control of this population during disease progression and ideally trying to inhibit their emergence during asymptomatic stages. AbAs expression of S100β at levels higher than wild type astrocytes may imply that they have a role in the amplification of the inflammatory response, therefore new anti-inflammatory drugs targeting the production of pro-inflammatory cytokines by a blockade of NFkB activation may have positive results, moreover because NFkB is downstream to S100β [54]. For example, FDA has been approved a drug called mitoxantrone for multiple sclerosis treatment because it inhibited production of IL-12 and IL-23 and suppressed the expression of C-reactive protein by astrocytes in culture and LPS induction of NFkB DNA-binding activity in primary astrocytes, suggesting a novel mechanism that suppresses the expression of astrocytic pro-inflammatory molecules helping to modulate inflammatory diseases [95]. However, as AbAs seem to loss S100β at higher passages, neuroprotection by targeting this via might be successful only during asymptomatic stages. Targeting neuroinflammation, recently, it has been shown that the tyrosine kinase inhibitor (masitinib) that is used to control cancer cell proliferation reduced the emergence of aberrant glial cells in the degenerating spinal cord of SOD1G93A paralytic rats and delay disease progression [87]. Authors proposed that masitinib acts preventing the appearance of aberrant glial phenotypes, likely through the inhibition of CSF-1R kinase which activation potentiates inflammatory phenotypes and glial reactivity, and that are particularly effective on proliferating but not on post-mitotic cells [96]. Furthermore, masitinib also prevented astrocyte-induced motor neuron death in cell cultures [97], suggesting that neuroprotection can be achieved through different pathways. In accordance, other report has shown that CSF-1R blockade with the drug GW2580 administered to ALS mice several weeks before paralysis onset decreased both microgliosis and slowed disease progression [98], thus opening a wider avenue to treat aberrant glial phenotypes. Finally, although molecular genetic techniques devoted to switch genes on or off, or to edit their nucleotide sequences, once developed and approved can be effective therapeutic tools to the inherited ALS forms, pharmacological approaches directed against aberrant glial phenotypes may help to control disease progression in a wider range of patients.

5. Conclusions

All data reviewed here suggest that aberrant astrocytes or more generally, aberrant glial cells, are among the most important players in CNS damage causing deleterious effects through many potential patho-mechanisms, mostly sustained on their exacerbated proliferation together with their unprecedented neurotoxicity. Therefore, controlling these populations seems at least equally important than maintenance or restoration of homeostatic astrocyte functions to achieve CNS protection and repair. Moreover, AbAs seemed a better pharmacological target than astrocytes, since therapeutic approaches focused on astrocytes have to be carefully tailored taking into account their multiple faces, moreover in the context of neurodegeneration where several cell types are involved. Future investigation should aim to elucidate if AbAs can indeed be feasible targets to avoid initiation, progression or outcome of neurodegeneration.

Acknowledgements

We thank IIBCE (MEC), PEDECIBA, and UdelaR, URUGUAY.

Conflict of interest

There is no conflict of interest.

Author details

Gabriel Otero Damianovich[1], Olga Cristina Parada[2], Pablo Díaz-Amarilla[1], Eugenia Eloísa Isasi[1,2], Carmen Isabel Bolatto Pereira[2] and Silvia Olivera-Bravo[1]*

1 Cell and Molecular Neurobiology, Institute of Biological Research Clemente Estable (IIBCE), Montevideo, Uruguay

2 Department of Histology and Embriology, School of Medicine (UdelaR), Montevideo, Uruguay

*Address all correspondence to: solivera@iibce.edu.uy

References

[1] Cleveland DW, Rothstein JD. From Charcot to Lou Gehrig: Deciphering selective motor neuron death in ALS. Nature Reviews Neuroscience. 2001;**2**:806-819. DOI: 10.1038/35097565

[2] Kiernan MC, Vucic S, Cheah BC, Turner MR, Eisen A, Hardiman O, et al. Amyotrophic lateral sclerosis. Lancet. 2011;**377**(9769):942-955. DOI: 10.1016/S0140-6736(10)61156-7

[3] Pehar M, Harlan BA, Killoy KM, Vargas MR. Role and therapeutic potential of astrocytes in amyotrophic lateral sclerosis. Current Pharmaceutical Design. 2017;**23**(33):5010-5021. DOI: 10.2174/1381612823666170622095802

[4] Ilieva H, Maragakis NJ. Motoneuron disease: Basic science. In: Beart P, Robinson M, Rattray M, Maragakis NJ, editors. Advances in Neurobiology 15; Neurodegenerative Diseases Pathology, Mechanisms, and Potential Therapeutic Targets. Cham: Springer; 2017. pp. 163-190. DOI: 10.1007/978-3-319-57193-5

[5] Al-Chalabi A, Fang F, Hanby MF, Leigh PN, Shaw CE, Ye W, et al. An estimate of amyotrophic lateral sclerosis heritability using twin data. Journal of Neurology, Neurosurgery, and Psychiatry. 2010;**81**(12):1324-1326. DOI: 10.1136/jnnp.2010.207464

[6] Cudkowicz ME, Warren L, Francis JW, Lloyd KJ, Friedlander RM, Borges LF, et al. Intrathecal administration of recombinant human superoxide dismutase 1 in amyotrophic lateral sclerosis: A preliminary safety and pharmacokinetic study. Neurology. 1997;**49**:213-222. DOI: 10.1212/WNL.49.1.213

[7] Rosen DR. Mutations in Cu/Zn superoxide dismutase gene are associated with familial amyotrophic lateral sclerosis. Nature. 1993;**364**:362. DOI: 10.1038/362059a0

[8] Neumann M, Sampathu DM, Kwong LK, Truax AC, Micsenyi MC, Chou TT, et al. Ubiquitinated TDP-43 in frontotemporal lobar degeneration and amyotrophic lateral sclerosis. Science. 2006;**314**(5796):130-133. DOI: 10.1126/science.1134108

[9] Kwiatkowski TJ Jr, Bosco DA, Leclerc AL, Tamrazian E, Vanderburg CR, Russ C, et al. Mutations in the FUS/TLS gene on chromosome 16 cause familial amyotrophic lateral sclerosis. Science. 2009;**323**(5918):1205-1208. DOI: 10.1126/science.1166066

[10] Vance C, Rogelj B, Hortobágyi T, De Vos KJ, Nishimura AL, Sreedharan J, et al. Mutations in FUS, an RNA processing protein, cause familial amyotrophic lateral sclerosis type 6. Science. 2009;**323**(5918):1208-1211. DOI: 10.1126/science.1165942

[11] Todd PK, Paulson HL. RNA-mediated neurodegeneration in repeat expansion disorders. Annals of Neurology. 2010;**67**(3):291-300. DOI: 10.1002/ana.21948

[12] Ling SC, Polymenidou M, Cleveland DW. Converging mechanisms in ALS and FTD: Disrupted RNA and protein homeostasis. Neuron. 2013;**79**(3):416-438. DOI: 10.1016/j.neuron.2013.07.033

[13] van Blitterswijk M, DeJesus-Hernandez M, Rademakers R. How do C9ORF72 repeat expansions cause amyotrophic lateral sclerosis and frontotemporal dementia: Can we learn from other noncoding repeat expansion disorders? Current Opinion in Neurology. 2012;**25**(6):689-700. DOI: 10.1097/WCO.0b013e32835a3efb

[14] Mori K, Weng SM, Arzberger T, May S, Rentzsch K, Kremmer E, et al. The C9orf72 GGGGCC repeat is translated into aggregating dipeptide repeat proteins in FTLD/ALS. Science. 2013;**339**(6125):1335-1338. DOI: 10.1126/science.1232927

[15] Ash PE, Bieniek KF, Gendron TF, Caulfield T, Lin WL, Dejesus-Hernandez M, et al. Unconventional translation of C9ORF72 GGGGCC expansion generates insoluble polypeptides specific to c9FTD/ALS. Neuron. 2013;**77**(4):639-646. DOI: 10.1016/j.neuron.2013.02.004

[16] Sulston JE, Horvitz HR. Post-embryonic cell lineages of the nematode, Caenorhabditis elegans. Developmental Biology. 1977;**56**(1):110-156. DOI: 10.1016/0012-1606(77)90158-0

[17] Howe K, Clark MD, Torroja CF, Torrance J, Berthelot C, Muffato M, et al. The zebrafish reference genome sequence and its relationship to the human genome. Nature. 2013;**496**(7446):498-503. DOI: 10.1038/nature12111

[18] Gurney ME, Pu H, Chiu AY, Dal Canto MC, Polchow CY, Alexander DD, et al. Motor neuron degeneration in mice that express a human Cu, Zn superoxide dismutase mutation. Science. 1994;**264**:1772-1775. DOI: 10.1126/science.8209258

[19] Howland DS, Liu J, She Y, Goad B, Maragakis NJ, Kim B, et al. Focal loss of the glutamate transporter EAAT2 in a transgenic rat model of SOD1 mutant-mediated amyotrophic lateral sclerosis (ALS). Proceedings of the National Academy of Sciences of the United States of America. 2002;**99**:1604-1609. DOI: 10.1073/pnas.032539299

[20] Turner BJ, Talbot K. Transgenics, toxicity and therapeutics in rodent models of mutant SOD1 mediated familial ALS. Progress in Neurobiology. 2008;**85**:94-134. DOI: 10.1016/j.pneurobio.2008.01.001

[21] Yamanaka K, Chun SJ, Boillee S, Fujimori-Tonou N, Yamashita H, Gutmann DH, et al. Astrocytes as determinants of disease progression in inherited amyotrophic lateral sclerosis. Nature Neuroscience. 2008;**11**(3):251-253. DOI: 10.1038/nn2047

[22] Boillée S, Vande Velde C, Cleveland DW. ALS: A disease of motor neurons and their non neuronal neighbors. Neuron. 2006;**52**:39-59. DOI: 10.3109/21678421.2013.778548

[23] Ilieva H, Polymenidou M, Cleveland DW. Non-cell autonomous toxicity in neurodegenerative disorders: ALS and beyond. The Journal of Cell Biology. 2009;**187**:761-772. DOI: 10.1083/jcb.200908164

[24] Cassina P, Cassina A, Pehar M, Castellanos R, Gandelman M, de León A, et al. Mitochondrial dysfunction in SOD1G93A-bearing astrocytes promotes motor neuron degeneration: Prevention by mitochondrial-targeted antioxidants. The Journal of Neuroscience. 2008;**28**:4115-4122. DOI: 10.1523/JNEUROSCI.5308-07.2008

[25] Di Giorgio FP, Boulting GL, Bobrowicz S, Eggan KC. Human embryonic stem cell-derived motor neurons are sensitive to the toxic effect of glial cells carrying an ALS-causing mutation. Cell Stem Cell. 2008;**3**:637-648. DOI: 10.1016/j.stem.2008.09.017

[26] Nagai M, Re DB, Nagata T, Chalazonitis A, Jessell TM, Wichterle H, et al. Astrocytes expressing ALS-linked mutated SOD1 release factors selectively toxic to motor neurons. Nature Neuroscience. 2007;**10**:615-622. DOI: 10.1038/nn1876

[27] Haidet-Phillips AM, Hester ME, Miranda CJ, Meyer K, Braun L, Frakes A, et al. Astrocytes from familial and sporadic ALS patients are toxic to motor neurons. Nature Biotechnology. 2011;**29**:824-828. DOI: 10.1038/nbt.1957

[28] Re DB, Le Verche V, Yu C, Amoroso MW, Politi KA, Phani S, et al. Necroptosis drives motor neuron death in models of both sporadic and familial ALS. Neuron. 2014;**81**:1001-1008. DOI: 10.1016/j.neuron.2014.01.011

[29] Wegorzewska I, Bell S, Cairns NJ, Miller TM, Baloh RH. TDP-43 mutant transgenic mice develop features of ALS and frontotemporal lobar degeneration. Proceedings of the National Academy of Sciences of the United States of America. 2009;**106**(44):18809-18814. DOI: 10.1073/pnas.0908767106

[30] Swarup V, Phaneuf D, Bareil C, Robertson J, Rouleau GA, Kriz J, et al. Pathological hallmarks of amyotrophic lateral sclerosis/frontotemporal lobar degeneration in transgenic mice produced with TDP-43 genomic fragments. Brain. 2011;**134**(9): 2610-2626. DOI: 10.1093/brain/awr159

[31] Maragakis NJ, Rothstein JD. Mechanisms of disease: Astrocytes in neurodegenerative disease. Nature Clinical Practice. Neurology. 2006;**2**(12):679-689. DOI: 10.1038/ncpneuro0355

[32] Sofroniew MV, Vinters HV. Astrocytes: Biology and pathology. Acta Neuropathologica. 2010;**119**(1): 7-35. DOI: 10.1007/s00401-009-0619-8

[33] Verkhratsky A, Sofroniew MV, Messing A, de Lanerolle NC, Rempe D, Rodríguez JJ, et al. Neurological diseases as primary gliopathies: A reassessment of neurocentrism. ASN Neuro. 2012;**4**(3):e00082. DOI: 10.1042/AN20120010

[34] Sloan SA, Barres BA. Mechanisms of astrocyte development and their contributions to neurodevelopmental disorders. Current Opinion in Neurobiology. 2014;**27**:75-81. DOI: 10.1016/j.conb.2014.03.005

[35] Barbeito LH, Pehar M, Cassina P, Vargas MR, Peluffo H, Viera L, et al. A role for astrocytes in motor neuron loss in amyotrophic lateral sclerosis. Brain Research. Brain Research Reviews. 2004;**47** (1-3):263-274. DOI: 10.1016/j.brainresrev.2004.05.003

[36] Hostenbach S, Cambron M, D'haeseleer M, Kooijman R, De Keyser J. Astrocyte loss and astrogliosis in neuroinflammatory disorders. Neuroscience Letters. 2014;**565**:39-41. DOI: 10.1016/j.neulet.2013.10.012

[37] Pekny M, Wilhelmsson U, Pekna M. The dual role of astrocyte activation and reactive gliosis. Neuroscience Letters. 2014;**565**:30-38. DOI: 10.1016/j.neulet.2013.12.071

[38] Olivera-Bravo S, Isasi E, Fernández A, Casanova G, Rosillo JC, Barbeito L. Astrocyte dysfunction in developmental neurometabolic diseases. Advances in Experimental Medicine and Biology. 2016;**949**:227-243. DOI: 10.1007/978-3-319-40764-7_11

[39] Kuno R, Yoshida Y, Nitta A, Nabeshima T, Wang J, Sonobe Y, et al. The role of TNF-alpha and its receptors in the production of NGF and GDNF by astrocytes. Brain Research. 2006;**1116**(1):12-18. DOI: 10.1016/j.brainres.2006.07.120

[40] Díaz-Amarilla P, Olivera-Bravo S, Trias E, Cragnolini A, Martínez-Palma L, Cassina P, et al. Phenotypically aberrant astrocytes that promote motoneuron damage in a model of inherited amyotrophic lateral sclerosis. Proceedings of the National Academy of Sciences of the United States of

America. 2011;**108**:18126-18131. DOI: 10.1073/pnas.1110689108

[41] Jiménez-Riani M, Díaz-Amarilla P, Isasi E, Casanova G, Barbeito L, Olivera-Bravo S. Ultrastructural features of aberrant glial cells isolated from the spinal cord of paralytic rats expressing the amyotrophic lateral sclerosis-linked SOD1G93A mutation. Cell and Tissue Research. 2017;**370**(3):391-401. DOI: 10.1007/s00441-017-2681-1

[42] Yoshiyama Y, Zhang B, Bruce J, Trojanowski JQ, Lee VMY. Reduction of detyrosinated microtubules and Golgi fragmentation are linked to tau-induced degeneration in astrocytes. The Journal of Neuroscience. 2003;**23**:10662-10671. DOI: 10.1523/JNEUROSCI.23-33-10662.2003

[43] Kawamata H, Manfredi G. Mitochondrial dysfunction and intracellular calcium dysregulation in ALS. Mechanisms of Ageing and Development. 2010;**131**:517-526. DOI: 10.1016/j.mad.2010.05.003

[44] Sasaki S, Iwata M. Dendritic synapses of anterior horn neurons in amyotrophic lateral sclerosis: An ultrastructural study. Acta Neuropathologica. 2006;**91**:278-283. DOI: 10.1016/0304-3940(96)12314-4

[45] Gallagher CM, Walter P. Ceapins inhibit ATF6a signaling by selectively preventing transport of ATF6a to the Golgi apparatus during ER stress. eLife. 2016;**5**:e11880. DOI: 10.7554/eLife.11880

[46] Hetz C, Thielen P, Matus S, Nassif M, Court F, Kiffin R, et al. XBP-1 deficiency in the nervous system protects against amyotrophic lateral sclerosis by increasing autophagy. Genes & Development. 2009;**23**:2294-2306. DOI: 10.1101/gad.1830709

[47] Kondo S, Murakami T, Tatsumi K, Ogata M, Kanemoto S, Otori K, et al. OASIS, a CREB/ATF-family member, modulates UPR signalling in astrocytes. Nature Cell Biology. 2005;**7**:186-194. DOI: 10.1038/ncb1213

[48] Hur YS, Kim KD, Paek SH. Yoo SH (2010) evidence for the existence of secretory granule (dense-core vesicle)-based inositol 1,4,5-trisphosphate-dependent Ca^{2+} signaling system in astrocytes. PLoS ONE. 2010;**5**(8):e11973. DOI: 10.1371/journal.pone.0011973

[49] Ozawa H, Takata K. The Granin family-its role in sorting and secretory granule formation. Cell Structure and Function. 1995;**20**:415-420. DOI: 10.1247/csf.20.415

[50] Kabeya Y, Mizushima N, Ueno T, Yamamoto A, Kirisako T, Noda T, et al. LC3, a mammalian homologue of yeast Apg8p, is localized in autophagosome membranes after processing. The EMBO Journal. 2000;**19**:5720-5728. DOI: 10.1093/emboj/19.21.5720

[51] Herrera F, Martin V, Carrera P, García-Santos G, Rodriguez-Blanco J, Rodriguez C, et al. Tryptamine induces cell death with ultrastructural features of autophagy in neurons and glia: Possible relevance for neurodegenerative disorders. The Anatomical Record. 2006;**288**:1026-1030. DOI: 10.1002/ar.a.20368

[52] Robert F, Hervor TK. Abnormal organelles in cultured astrocytes are largely enhanced by streptomycin and intensively by gentamicin. Neuroscience. 2007;**144**:191-197. DOI: 10.1016/j.neuroscience.2006.08.059

[53] Nixon RA, Wegiel J, Kumar A, Yu WH, Peterhoff C, Cataldo A, et al. Extensive involvement of autophagy in Alzheimer disease: An immuno-electron microscopy study. Journal of Neuropathology and Experimental Neurology. 2005;**64**:113-122. DOI: 10.1093/jnen/64.2.113

[54] Donato R, Sorci G, Riuzzi F, Arcuri C, Bianchi R, Brozzi F, et al. S100B's double life: Intracellular regulator and extracellular signal. Biochimica et Biophysica Acta. 2009;**1793**(6):1008-1022. DOI: 10.1016/j.bbamcr.2008.11.009

[55] Gonzalez-Reyes RE, Rubiano MG. Astrocyte's RAGE: More than just a question of mood. Central Nervous System Agents in Medicinal Chemistry. 2018;**18**(1):39-48. DOI: 10.2174/1871524916999160505105121

[56] Fife CM, McCarroll JA, Kavallaris M. Movers and shakers: Cell cytoskeleton in cancer metastasis. British Journal of Pharmacology. 2014;**171**(24):5507-5523. DOI: 10.1111/bph.12704

[57] Schmitt F, Hussain G, Dupuis L, Loeffler JP, Henriques A. A plural role for lipids in motor neuron diseases: Energy, signaling and structure. Frontiers in Cellular Neuroscience. 2014;**8**:25. DOI: 10.3389/fncel.2014.00025. eCollection 2014

[58] Taylor JP, Brown RH Jr, Cleveland DW. Decoding ALS: From genes to mechanism. Nature. 2016;**539**:197-206. DOI: 10.1038/nature20413

[59] Valenzuela V, Oñate M, Hetz C, Court FA. Injury to the nervous system: A look into the ER. Brain Research. 2016;**1648**: 617-625. DOI: 10.1016/j.brainres.2016.04.053

[60] Walter P, Ron D. The unfolded protein response: From stress pathway to homeostatic regulation. Science. 2011;**334**:1081-1086. DOI: 10.1126/science.1209038

[61] Oakes SA, Papa FR. The role of endoplasmic reticulum stress in human pathology. Annual Review of Pathology.2015;**10**: 173-194. DOI: 10.1146/annurev-pathol-012513-104649

[62] Halliday M, Mallucci GR. Modulating the unfolded protein response to prevent neurodegeneration and enhance memory. Neuropathology and Applied Neurobiology. 2015;**41**: 414-427. DOI: 10.1111/nan.12211

[63] Lee S, Shang Y, Redmond SA, Urisman A, Tang AA, Li KH, et al. Activation of HIPK2 promotes ER stress-mediated neurodegeneration in amyotrophic lateral sclerosis. Neuron. 2016;**91**:41-55. DOI: 10.1016/j.neuron.2016.05.021

[64] Suzuki H, Matsuoka M. TDP-43 toxicity is mediated by the unfolded protein response-unrelated induction of C/EBP homologous protein expression. Journal of Neuroscience Research. 2012;**90**:641-647. DOI: 10.1002/jnr.22777

[65] Tsang KY, Chan D, Bateman JF, Cheah KSE. In vivo cellular adaptation to ER stress: Survival strategies with double-edged consequences. Journal of Cell Science. 2010;**123**:2145-2154. DOI: 10.1242/jcs.068833

[66] Walker AK, Soo KY, Sundaramoorthy V, Parakh S, Ma Y, Farg MA, et al. ALS-associated TDP-43 induces endoplasmic reticulum stress, which drives cytoplasmic TDP-43 accumulation and stress granule formation. PLoS ONE. 2013;**8**(11):e81170. DOI: 10.1371/journal.pone.0081170

[67] Pennetta G, Welte MA. Emerging links between lipid droplets and motor neuron diseases. Developmental Cell. 2018;**45**:427-432. DOI: 10.1016/j.devcel.2018.05.002

[68] Ernst WL, Shome K, Wu CC, Gong X, Frizzell RA, Aridor M. VAMP-associated proteins (VAP) as receptors that couple cystic fibrosis transmembrane conductance regulator (CFTR) proteostasis with lipid homeostasis. The Journal of Biological

Chemistry. 2016;**291**:5206-5220. DOI: 10.1074/jbc.M115.692749

[69] Janer A, Martin E, Muriel MP, Latouche M, Fujigasaki H, Ruberg M, et al. PML clastosomes prevent nuclear accumulation of mutant ataxin-7 and other polyglutamine proteins. The Journal of Cell Biology. 2006;**174**(1):65-76. DOI: 10.1074/jbc.M115.692749

[70] Zhu L, Brangwynne CP. Nuclear bodies: The emerging biophysics of nucleoplasmic phases. Current Opinion in Cell Biology. 2015;**34**:23-30. DOI: 10.1016/j.ceb.2015.04.003

[71] Seilhean D, Takahashi J, El Hachimi KH, Fujigasaki H, Lebre AS, Biancalana V, et al. Amyotrophic lateral sclerosis with neuronal intranuclear protein inclusions. Acta Neuropathologica. 2004;**108**:81-87. DOI: 10.1007/s00401-004-0855-x

[72] Welte MA. Expanding roles for lipid droplets. Current Biology. 2015;**25**:470-481. DOI: 10.1016/j.cub.2015.04.004

[73] Stallings NR, Puttaparthi K, Dowling KJ, Luther CM, Burns DK, Davis K, et al. TDP-43, an ALS linked protein, regulates fat deposition and glucose homeostasis. PLoS ONE. 2013;**8**:e71793. DOI: 10.1371/journal.pone.0071793

[74] Chiang PM, Ling J, Jeong YH, Price DL, Aja SM, Wong PC. Deletion of TDP-43 down-regulates Tbc1d1, a gene linked to obesity, and alters body fat metabolism. Proceedings of the National Academy of Sciences of the United States of America. 2010;**107**(37):16320-16324. DOI: 10.1073/pnas.1002176107

[75] Miyazaki K, Masamoto K, Morimoto N, Kurata T, Mimoto T, Obata T, et al. Early and progressive impairment of spinal blood flow-glucose metabolism coupling in motor neuron degeneration of ALS model mice. Journal of Cerebral Blood Flow and Metabolism. 2012;**32**(3):456-467. DOI: 10.1038/jcbfm.2011.155

[76] Liu L, Zhang K, Sandoval H, Yamamoto S, Jaiswal M, Sanz E, et al. Glial lipid droplets and ROS induced by mitochondrial defects promote neurodegeneration. Cell. 2015;**160**:177-190. DOI: 10.1016/j.cell.2014.12.019

[77] Yamamoto S, Jaiswal M, Charng WL, Gambin T, Karaca E, Mirzaa G, et al. A drosophila genetic resource of mutants to study mechanisms underlying human genetic diseases. Cell. 2014;**159**:200-214. DOI: 10.1016/j.cell.2014.09.002

[78] Li YR, King OD, Shorter J, Gitler AD. Stress granules as crucibles of ALS pathogenesis. The Journal of Cell Biology. 2013;**201**:361-372. DOI: 10.1083/jcb.201302044

[79] Urushitani M, Ezzi SA, Matsuo A, Tooyama I, Julien JP. The endoplasmic reticulum-Golgi pathway is a target for translocation and aggregation of mutant superoxide dismutase linked to ALS. The FASEB Journal. 2006;**22**:2476-2487. DOI: 10.1096/fj.07-092783

[80] Eagle H, Levine EM. Growth regulatory effects of cellular interaction. Nature. 1967;**213**:1102-1106. DOI: 10.1038/2131102a0

[81] Choi EH, Dai Y. SIRT1 controls cell proliferation by regulating contact inhibition. Biochemical and Biophysical Research Communications. 2016;**478**(2):868-872. DOI: 10.1016/j.bbrc.2016.08.041

[82] Yang C, Iyer RR, Yu AC, Yong RL, Park DM, Weil RJ, et al. β-Catenin signaling initiates the activation of astrocytes and its dysregulation contributes to the pathogenesis

of astrocytomas. Proceedings of the National Academy of Sciences of the United States of America. 2012;**109**:6963-6968. DOI: 10.1073/pnas.1118754109

[83] Baker DJ, Blackburn DJ, Keatinge M, Sokhi D, Viskaitis P, Heath PR, et al. Lysosomal and phagocytic activity is increased in astrocytes during disease progression in the SOD1G93A mouse model of amyotrophic lateral sclerosis. Frontiers in Cellular Neuroscience. 2015;**9**:410. DOI: 10.3389/fncel.2015.00410

[84] Das MM, Svendsen CN. Astrocytes show reduced support of motor neurons with aging that is accelerated in a rodent model of ALS. Neurobiology of Aging. 2015;**36**:1130-1139. DOI: 10.1016/j.neurobiolaging.2014.09.020

[85] Song SW, Miranda CJ, Braun L, Meyer K, Frakes AE, Ferraiuolo L, et al. MHC class I protects motor neurons from astrocyte-induced toxicity in amyotrophic lateral sclerosis (ALS). Nature Medicine. 2016;**22**:397-403. DOI: 10.1038/nm.4052

[86] Trias E, Díaz-Amarilla P, Olivera-Bravo S, Isasi E, Drechsel DA, Lopez N, et al. Phenotypic transition of microglia into astrocyte-like cells associated with disease onset in a model of inherited ALS. Frontiers in Cellular Neuroscience. 2013;7:274. DOI: 10.3389/fncel.2013.00274

[87] Trias E, Ibarburu S, Barreto-Núñez R, Babdor J, Maciel TT, Guillo M, et al. Post-paralysis tyrosine kinase inhibition with masitinib abrogates neuroinflammation and slows disease progression in inherited amyotrophic lateral sclerosis. Journal of Neuroinflammation. 2016;**13**(1):177. DOI: 10.1186/s12974-016-0620-9

[88] Lamp J, Keyser B, Koeller DM, Ullrich K, Braulke T, Mühlhausen C. Glutaric aciduria type 1 metabolites impair the succinate transport from astrocytic to neuronal cells. The Journal of Biological Chemistry. 2011;**286**(20):17777-17784. DOI: 10.1074/jbc.M111.232744

[89] Miquel E, Cassina A, Martínez-Palma L, Souza JM, Bolatto C, Rodríguez-Bottero S, et al. Neuroprotective effects of the mitochondria-targeted antioxidant MitoQ in a model of inherited amyotrophic lateral sclerosis. Free Radical Biology & Medicine. 2014;**70**:204-213. DOI: 10.1016/j.freeradbiomed.2014.02.019

[90] Díaz-Amarilla P, Miquel E, Trostchansky A, Trias E, Ferreira AM, Freeman BA, et al. Electrophilic nitro-fatty acids prevent astrocyte-mediated toxicity to motor neurons in a cell model of familial amyotrophic lateral sclerosis via nuclear factor erythroid 2-related factor activation. Free Radical Biology & Medicine. 2016;**95**:112-120. DOI: 10.1016/j.freeradbiomed.2016.03.013

[91] Martínez-Palma L, Miquel E, Lagos-Rodríguez V, Barbeito L, Cassina A, Cassina P. Mitochondrial modulation by dichloroacetate reduces toxicity of aberrant glial cells and gliosis in the SOD1G93A rat model of amyotrophic lateral sclerosis. Neurotherapeutics. 2018;**16**(1):203-215. DOI: 10.1007/s13311-018-0659-7

[92] Miller RG, Mitchell JD, Moore DH. Riluzole for amyotrophic lateral sclerosis (ALS)/motor neuron disease (MND). Cochrane Database of Systematic Reviews. 2012;**14**(3):CD001447. DOI: 10.1002/14651858.CD001447.pub3

[93] Writing Group. Edaravone (MCI-186) ALS 19 Study Group. Safety and efficacy of edaravone in well defined patients with amyotrophic lateral sclerosis: A randomised, double-blind, placebo-controlled trial. Lancet

Neurology. 2017;**16**(7):505-512. DOI: 10.1016/S1474-4422(17)30115-1

[94] Scott A. On the treatment trail for ALS. Nature. 2017;**550**(7676):S120-S121. DOI: 10.1038/550S120a

[95] Burns SA, Lee Archer R, Chavis JA, Tull CA, Hensley LL, Drew PD. Mitoxantrone repression of astrocyte activation: Relevance to multiple sclerosis. Brain Research. 2012;**1473**:236-241. DOI: 10.1016/j.brainres.2012.07.054

[96] Kocic I, Kowianski P, Rusiecka I, Lietzau G, Mansfield C, Moussy A, et al. Neuroprotective effect of masitinib in rats with postischemic stroke. Naunyn-Schmiedeberg's Archives of Pharmacology. 2015;**388**(1):79-86. DOI: 10.1007/s00210-014-1061-6

[97] Rojas F, Gonzalez D, Cortes N, Ampuero E, Hernandez DE, Fritz E, et al. Reactive oxygen species trigger motoneuron death in non-cell-autonomous models of ALS through activation of c-Abl signaling. Frontiers in Cellular Neuroscience. 2015;**9**:203. DOI: 10.3389/fncel.2015.00203

[98] Martínez-Muriana A, Mancuso R, Francos-Quijorna I, Olmos-Alonso A, Osta R, Perry VH, et al. CSF1R blockade slows the progression of amyotrophic lateral sclerosis by reducing microgliosis and invasion of macrophages into peripheral nerves. Scientific Reports. 2016;**6**:25663. DOI: 10.1038/srep25663

Chapter 3

Stem Cell Therapy in Motor Neuron Disease

Alok Sharma, Hemangi Sane, Nandini Gokulchandran, Prerna Badhe, Amruta Paranjape, Radhika Pradhan, Rohit Das and Hema Biju

Abstract

Motor neuron disease (MND) is an insidious, fatal disorder that progresses with the selective loss of anterior horn cells of the spinal column. Over 150 years since it was first described, various therapeutic approaches have been tested in the quest of a cure but with little success. Current standard therapy only improves lifespan by a few months; palliative care is the only option available for patients. Stem cell therapy is a potent approach for the treatment of this devastating disease. A multitude of vitalizing effects, both paracrine and somatic, a robust safety profile, as well as ease of availability make a strong case for using these cells for therapeutic purposes. Coupled with rigorous rehabilitation, this powerful treatment modality has been shown to slow disease progression, improve quality of life, and increase survival, along with being well tolerated by amyotrophic lateral sclerosis (ALS)/MND patients. Compelling preclinical as well as clinical evidence abounds that stem cells hold great potential as a therapy for ALS/MND. Although not a definitive solution yet, stem cells have been verified to have slowed and/or halted disease progression in a subset of ALS/MND patients.

Keywords: motor neuron disease (MND), amyotrophic lateral sclerosis (ALS), stem cells, stem cell therapy, neurorehabilitation, neuro-regenerative rehabilitation therapy (NRRT), bone marrow-derived stem cells (BMSCs), bone marrow-derived mononuclear cells (BMMNCs)

1. Introduction

Motor neuron disease (MND) is a set of heterogeneous, idiopathic neurodegenerative syndromes characterized by progressive degeneration of anterior horn cells of the spinal cord, clinically characterized by weak and wasting musculature, which is eventually fatal [1]. Diagnosis is confirmed via thorough neuro-electrophysiological investigations [2]. Crude incidence of ALS/MND is 1.75 (1.55–1.96)/100,000 person-years of follow-up [3]. The male/female ratio is reported to be between 1 and 3 but varies with population and age [4]. The pathophysiology is multifarious (see Section 3.1), causing poor prognosis to be the major hurdle faced by clinicians worldwide [5]. Multidisciplinary symptomatic management is the sole option that can be availed by patients [6]. Pharmacological treatment includes riluzole (glutamate inhibition) [7], edaravone (effective only in the early stages) [8], and

Nuedexta (for treating pseudobulbar affect) [9]. Multidisciplinary rehabilitation is a key in managing secondary complications of the disease [10–12].

Studies worldwide endorse the safety and efficacy of stem cells as a therapeutic intervention, for a variety of neurological disorders [13–15], including ALS/MND [16–22]. Stem cells are a potent weapon in the fight against neurodegeneration. These cells hold the unique capacity to self-renew indefinitely while also giving rise to differentiated progeny under defined physiological conditions, thus repopulating damaged tissue [23]. Exercise has also been shown to enhance the mobilization and recruitment of these cells [24]. Given these properties, harnessing the potential of stem cells as a therapy to attenuate disease progression for neurodegenerative disorders, along with customized rehabilitative regimes, has gained traction in recent years.

2. Stem cells

The defining characteristics [25] of a stem cell are the unique capabilities of the following:

2.1 Clonogenicity

Stem cells self-renew throughout life, i.e., the cells undergo symmetric division under defined physiological conditions to produce identical daughter cells and thereby maintain the stem cell pool in the organism.

2.2 Multilineage differentiation

Under certain physiological conditions, stem cells may differentiate and divide asymmetrically to yield an identical daughter cell and a nonidentical, specialized daughter cell that acquires the properties of a cell type specific to a tissue.

2.3 Tissue regeneration

Stem cells have the capacity to renew the tissues that they populate. The body contains stem cell "niches," i.e., specific regulatory microenvironments conducive to the maintenance, proliferation, and differentiation of stem cells [26].

Depending on the source, stem cells are classified as embryonic stem cells (ESCs), fetal stem cells (FSCs), adult stem cells (ASCs), and induced pluripotent stem cells (iPSCs). ASCs are further classified into bone marrow stem cells (BMSCs), umbilical cord stem cells (UCSCs), and adipose tissue-derived stem cells (ADSCs). ESCs are pluripotent, self-renewing cells derived from the inner mass of the preimplantation blastocyst [27]. Their most obvious benefit is their pluripotency. However, ESCs tend to be highly tumorigenic, require considerable manipulation, and are in the hotbed of ethical debates [28]. FSCs are multipotent cells obtained from fetal tissues of natural, spontaneous abortuses that undergo in utero death within a specific gestational age range [29]. Limited supply, high degree of heterogeneity in the cell viability and cellular composition, and ethical issues hamper their clinical application [30].

Among ASCs, BMSCs take the lead in stem cell therapy in a wide variety of neurological disorders owing to their robust safety profile and efficient integration into host parenchyma [31–33]. Because these are adult cells, these are easily available and are not tumorigenic. The distinctive advantage of the BMSCs over other cell types is the lack of ethical issues for acquisition and administration. Currently, these comprise the most widely employed therapeutic strategy [19, 22, 31, 34–36]. UCSCs overcome the ethical concerns faced by the ESCs due to the ease of collection postpartum and minimal processing while posing no risk for the mother or the child. These cells, however, lose their advantage due to slow engraftment, limited single-dose availability, and long-term storage issues. Hereditary disorders further limit the benefits of UCSCs [37]. A minimally invasive subcutaneous accessibility and isolation procedure and a robust, long-term proliferation capacity outline the ADSCs' superiority [38, 39]. However, these cells find their limits in the presence of a highly heterogeneous population [40]. Pluripotent stem cells generated from cultured adult skin fibroblast cells by "inducing" dedifferentiation of unipotent, differentiated adult tissue cells by the addition of only a few defined factors are known as induced pluripotent stem cells [41]. iPSCs circumvent ethical concerns over the use of human embryos for the generation of cells of a desired tissue. However, oncogenic factors are used for induction of iPSCs' phenotype and may risk spontaneous induction of cancerous phenotypes and genomic instability [42].

3. Stem cells and motor neuron degeneration

3.1 Neuropathology of ALS/MND

Grossly, ALS/MND patients exhibit spinal cord atrophy and, in some cases, atrophy of cerebral white and gray matter (**Figure 1**). Some patients who have concomitant frontotemporal dementia show presence of cortical atrophy in frontal and temporal cortex. Microscopically, this is characterized by demyelination and axonal loss (**Figure 2**) [43–51].

3.2 Mechanism of action of stem cells

The clinical outcomes observed in ALS/MND are currently postulated to be due to various paracrine and somatic mechanisms that render a neurotrophic effect in various neurodegenerative diseases (**Figure 3**).

3.2.1 Paracrine effects

Stem cells confer neuroprotection through various paracrine mechanisms. Depending on the cellular microenvironment, these cells secrete and regulate a plethora of neurotrophic factors that are essential for the nervous system, like nerve growth factor-β (NGF-β, critical for the development and maintenance of the nervous system [52]), ciliary neurotrophic factor (CNTF, promotes neurogenesis [53]),

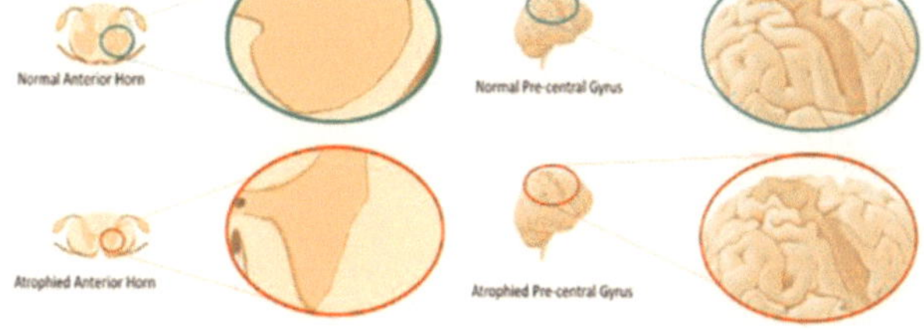

Figure 1.
The anterior horn of the spinal cord and the precentral gyrus are selectively affected and atrophy in ALS/MND.

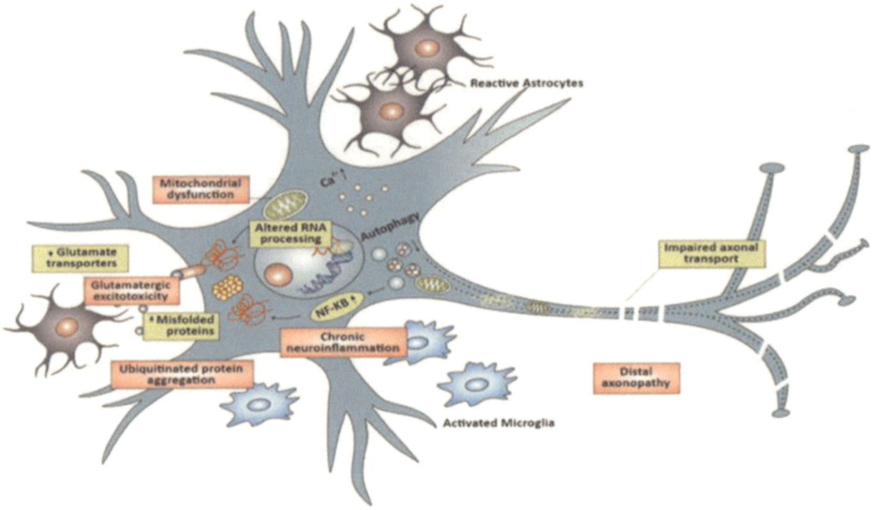

Figure 2.
Pathophysiology of motor neuron disease is multifaceted. Neuronal and nonneuronal cells like glial cell dysfunction have been postulated to contribute to the pathophysiology. Oxidative stress and subsequent rise in intracellular peroxidation, upregulation of astrocytic glutamate, mitochondrial abnormality, immune dysfunction, excitotoxicity, generalized neuroinflammation due secretion of pro-inflammatory cytokines by microglia, axonal transport system dysfunction, and synaptic failure are some of the mechanisms that have been identified. Apart from these mechanisms, abnormal cytoplasmic protein inclusions in patients with ALS have highlighted genetic causality.

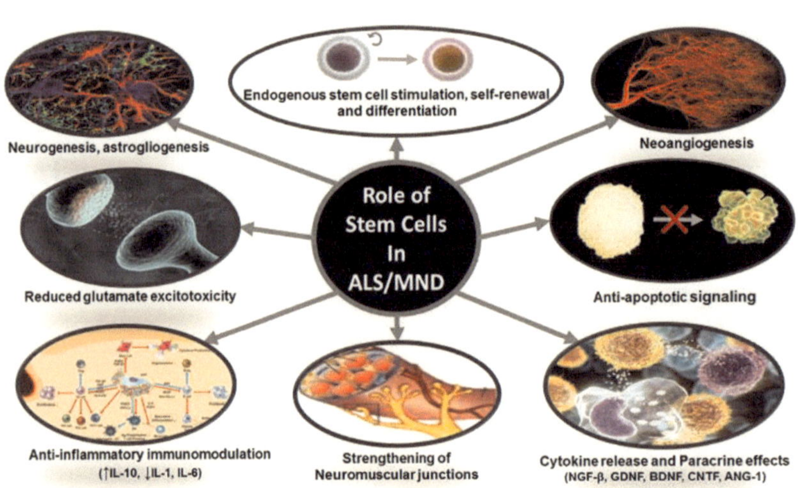

Figure 3.
Stem cells play multifarious roles in mitigating ALS/MND pathology.

brain-derived neurotrophic factor (BDNF, major role player in neuronal development as well as synaptic plasticity [53]), glial cell-derived neurotrophic factor (GDNF, plays an important role in striatal dopaminergic transport [54]), and angiopoietin 1 (ANG-1, promotes angiogenesis [55]).

3.2.2 Somatic effects

They also migrate to various tissues by homing strategies and have been shown to integrate into cells of target tissue.

3.2.3 Immunomodulation

These cells exude various beneficial immunomodulatory effects and are capable of homing onto injured sites, as guided by various chemoattractant pathways [55]. Modification of the exaggerated microglial response by immunomodulatory effects is also observed. Various secreted neurotrophic factors like connective tissue growth factor (CTGF), fibroblast growth factor (FGF) 2 and 7, and various interleukins (ILs) are responsible for cell proliferation and cytoprotection. Stem cells regulate innate and adaptive immune cells through release of soluble factors such as tumor growth factor (TGF)-β and elevation of regulatory T cells (Tregs) and T-helper-2 cells (Th2 cells) [56]. Reduced levels of TNF-α, IL-1β, IL-1α, and IL-6 and increased levels of IL-10 lead to an anti-inflammatory effect on the neural microenvironment [56–58], enhancing neuronal repair. Soluble factors from stem cells have been shown to significantly upregulate the expression of glutamate transporters in ALS astrocytes, resulting in enhanced glutamate uptake function. Stem cells also produce vascular endothelial growth factor (VEGF), hepatic growth factor (HGF), and insulin growth factor (IGF)-1, which are reported to have neuroprotective effects [57].

3.2.4 Neurogenesis

Mezey et al. have also shown that in a strain of mice incapable of developing cells of the myeloid and lymphoid lineages, transplanted adult bone marrow cells migrated into the brain and differentiated into cells that expressed neuron-specific antigens [58].

3.2.5 Oligodendrogenesis

Using cell fate tracking techniques, Sasaki and colleagues show that stem cells can differentiate into an oligodendroglial myelinating phenotype in vivo and repair demyelinated CNS [59].

3.2.6 Astrogliogenesis

Eglitis and Mezey have demonstrated the ability of hematopoietic stem cells (HSCs) to differentiate into both astrocytes and microglia in wild-type adult mice using in situ hybridization [60]. Wislet-Gendebien et al. show that nestin-positive (but not nestin-negative) mesenchymal stem cells are able to favor the astroglial lineage in certain stem cell progenitors. They also demonstrate that mesenchymal stem cells express leukemia inhibitory factor (LIF), CNTF, and BMP2 and BMP4 (bone morphogenic protein) mRNAs-cytokines known to play a role in astroglial fate decision [61].

3.2.7 Neoangiogenesis

Further secretion of growth factors like vascular endothelial growth factor (VEGF), fibroblast growth factor (FGF), and brain fibroblast growth factor (bFGF) leads to neoangiogenesis and upregulation of hormones like erythropoietin [62]. The cascade of events triggered due to these leads to formation of new vessels as well as improved blood circulation, thus retrieving lost tissue functions. Stem cells may thus be instrumental in arresting the disease progression through the abovementioned mechanisms.

4. Literature review

4.1 Preclinical studies

A wide variety of preclinical studies show that stem cells migrate to and restore lost function of damaged tissue in ALS/MND. Rodent studies have investigated different cell types such as mouse ES cells differentiated to neurons expressing green fluorescent protein (GFP) under the promoter of the motor neuron (MN)-specific gene hb9, mesenchymal stem cells (MSCs), human bone marrow mesenchymal stem cells (hMSCs) obtained from an ALS patient (ALS-hMSCs), human neural stem cells (hNSCs), human cord blood stem cells (HuCB-MNCs), human embryonic stem cell-derived motor neuron progenitors (hMNPs), bone marrow cells (BMCs), mesenchymal stromal (stem) cells (MSCs), human umbilical cord blood (MNC-hUCB), human fetal spinal neural stem cells (hNSCs), human iPSC-derived neural progenitors (hiPSNPs), HB1.F3.Olig2 cell (stable immortalized hNSCs encoding the OLIG2 gene)-derived motor neurons, human amniotic mesenchymal stem cells (hAMSCs), glial-rich neural progenitors derived from human iPSCs, enriched population of embryonic stem cell-derived astrocytes (hES-AS), and neural progenitor cells secreting GDNF ($hNPC^{GDNF}$) [63–79].

Primarily, stem cells have been shown to have a vast repertoire of paracrine effects, including release of neurotrophic factors such as GDNF, BDNF, vascular endothelial growth factor (VEGF), insulin-like growth factor (IGF)-1, NGF, and neurotrophin (NT)-3. Stem cells also confer neuroprotection by migrating, efficiently engrafting into target tissue, reducing astrogliosis, and differentiating into neuroglial cell types. Further, they improve motor performance as measured on rotarod (test measuring rodent balance, grip strength, endurance, and motor coordination), delay disease pathology, and safely extend survival in ALS rodent models (see Appendix) [20, 63–79].

A limitation of preclinical models of ALS, however, is the inherent inability to replicate the *sporadic* onset of ALS/MND, which constitutes majority of patients in clinical scenario [79]. Additionally, an obvious drawback is the underrepresentation of the genomic, anatomical, and physiological complexity of humans by the disease models, which may preclude the translation of results obtained in preclinical settings to the treatment of ALS patients.

4.2 Clinical studies

4.2.1 Worldwide published data

A systematic review and meta-analysis of clinical studies by Moura et al. [80] have suggested that stem cell therapy is a promising therapy and highlighted the need for studies with rigorous methodologies to better understand the efficacy of these therapies. **Table** 7 (see Appendix) summarizes the studies reviewed by Moura et al. and other studies that were published using stem cells as therapy in the past decade. Nineteen clinical studies are summarized; a variety of cells have been investigated in clinical settings, such as:

1. Autologous mesenchymal stem cells (intraspinal) [81]

2. Bone marrow-derived hematopoietic progenitor stem cells (intraspinal) [18]

3. Autologous peripheral blood stem (intracerebral) [82]

4. Autologous bone marrow stem cells (intrathecal) [83]

5. Autologous mesenchymal stem cells (intrathecal and intravenous) [31]

6. Olfactory ensheathing cells (intracerebral) and autologous mesenchymal stromal cells (intrathecal and intravenous or only intrathecal) [84]

7. Neural stem cells derived from a fetal spinal cord (intrathecal) [85]

8. Mesenchymal stem cells induced to secrete neurotrophic factors (intramuscular, intrathecal, or both) [86]

9. Autologous bone marrow stem cells (intraspinal) [34]

10. Autologous mesenchymal stem cells (intraspinal) [21]

11. Fetal olfactory ensheathing cells (intracerebral) [19]

12. Fetal-derived neural stem cells (intraspinal) [22]

13. NSI-566RSC (Neuralstem, Inc.), a human neural stem cell (intrathecal) [87]

14. Autologous bone marrow mononuclear cells (intrathecal) [16]

15. Mesenchymal stem cells (intrathecal) [35]

16. Autologous mesenchymal stem cells (intravenous, intrathecal) [88]

17. Autologous bone marrow stem cells (intramedullary) [89]

18. Autologous mesenchymal stem cells (intrathecal) [36]

Overwhelmingly, results point toward a robust safety profile for stem cell treatment in ALS/MND. Stem cell therapy has also proven to be efficacious in mitigating the hostility of a degenerating prognosis in all these studies (see Appendix). These data collectively advocate for the safety and efficacy of various types of stem cells for the treatment of this disease, although small scale; larger clinical trials with sufficient power are required for clearing the turbid field of ALS/MND therapy.

4.2.2 Our published results

4.2.2.1 Our published protocol for stem cell therapy in ALS/MND

4.2.2.1.1 Pre-intervention procedures

We use intrathecal autologous bone marrow mononuclear cell (BMMNC) transplantation for the treatment of ALS/MND, chosen according to the World Medical Association Declaration of Helsinki—Ethical Principles for Medical Research Involving Human Subjects. The ethical approval for the intervention is obtained from Institutional Ethics Committee (IEC). Our exclusion criteria include the presence of respiratory distress; thus, the effect of stem cell therapy on such patients cannot be assessed. Our inclusion criteria involve patients diagnosed as definite or probable ALS according to revised El Escorial criteria [90]. The procedure is explained to the patients in detail, and a written informed consent is obtained. Patients are thoroughly examined by an experienced team of doctors and therapists. Pre-surgical routine blood tests, urinalysis, and chest X-ray are carried out for assessing anesthetic and surgical fitness. About 300 μg of granulocyte colony-stimulating factor (G-CSF) injections are administrated subcutaneously 48 and 24 hours prior to BMMNC transplantation, as they enhance the mobility of BMMNCs, stimulates $CD34^+$ cells, and increases their survival as well as multiplication rate [91]. The transplant is then carried out in three steps (**Figure 4**).

4.2.2.1.2 Bone marrow aspiration

Performed in the operation theater under aseptic conditions, 100–120 ml of bone marrow is aspirated under local anesthesia from the region of anterior superior iliac spine and collected in the heparinized tubes.

4.2.2.1.3 Cell separation

Using density gradient centrifugation, stem cells are separated. The cell pellet is analyzed under a microscope using trypan blue to check for the viability of the cells. Cell number is counted using Tali cell counter. FACS analysis using CD34 PE antibody is used for identification of $CD34^+$ cells.

4.2.2.1.4 Cell transplantation

In the operation theater under aseptic conditions, the cells are transplanted intrathecally into the cerebrospinal fluid through lumbar puncture between the level of fourth and fifth lumbar vertebra, using an 18G Touhy needle.

4.2.2.1.5 Posttransplantation

Cell transplantation is followed by standard multidisciplinary rehabilitation including physiotherapy, occupational therapy, speech therapy, psychological intervention, aquatic therapy, and dietary advice. This approach is termed as neuro-regenerative rehabilitative therapy (NRRT). Standard medical treatment was continued with Rilutor. Tablet lithium was prescribed for 6 weeks for its neuroprotective properties. Lithium levels were monitored.

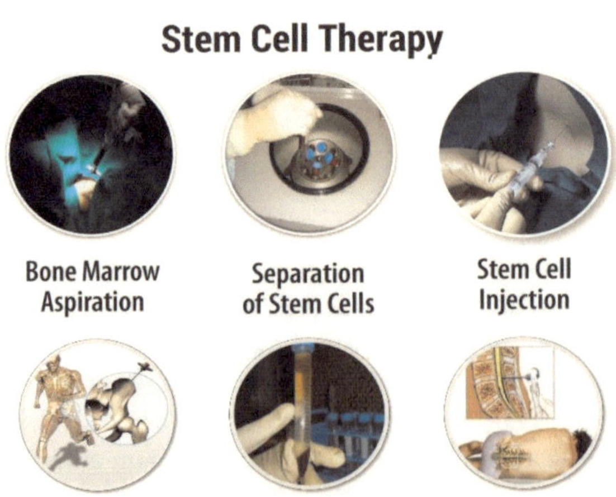

Figure 4.
Stem cell therapy protocol at NeuroGen Brain and Spine Institute.

4.2.2.2 Case series

We have published a retrospective controlled cohort study with a total of 57 ALS patients that investigates the effects of stem cell therapy, in addition to standard rehabilitation, lithium, and riluzole [79]. Out of these, 37 patients underwent autologous BMMNC transplantation, while the remaining 20 did not; these served as controls. We saw that there was a clinically significant difference of 30.38 months between the average survival duration of intervention and control groups. Intervention group survived for 87.76 (10.45) months, while controls survived for 57.38 (5.31) months. Patients with the onset of the disease below 50 years of age survived significantly longer ($p = 0.039$), while limb symptom onset and co-administration of lithium improved survival duration in a clinically significant manner [16]. Lithium increases the survival, potency, and target tissue integration of BMSCs [92]. It has been shown to confer neuroprotection in vitro by enhancing cellular BDNF [93]. In vivo, lithium has been shown to activate autophagy, normalize mitochondrial aberration, and suppress reactive astrogliosis. It also reduces ubiquitinated protein aggregates and increases the number of spared motor neurons in transgenic ALS mice [94]. Further, lithium is well tolerated by ALS patients who are on riluzole, even though it may not be effective by itself for treating ALS. This was confirmed by two trials: a phase III multicenter, randomized, double-blind, placebo-controlled trial (LiCALS) by Al-Chalabi et al. [95] and a phase IIb randomized, double-blind, placebo-controlled, sequential trial by Verstraete et al. [96]. Taken together, these results suggest that a combination strategy of stem cells and lithium may have played a pronounced role in the outcomes of this study, summarizes the prognostic factors that influence survival in the intervention group. Younger age at symptom onset and spinal symptom onset favors longer survival durations according to our findings. Post intervention, lithium prescription combined with standard riluzole treatment and comprehensive rehabilitation enhances the effect of cellular therapy (**Figure 5** and **Table 1**).

4.2.2.3 Case reports

A 40-year-old female suffering from ALS for 3 years was given intrathecal autologous BMMNC transplantation along with riluzole, lithium, and intensive rehabilitation. The disease progression slowed over 17 months along with improvements in neurological symptoms. de Carvalho et al. have previously reported that the ALSFRS-R score deteriorates about 17% every 6 months [97]; here, the ALSFRS-R score dropped only by 8% over 17 months after cell transplantation (**Figure 6** and **Table 2**) [98].

A 41-year-old female suffering from ALS for 3 years was given intrathecal autologous BMMNC therapy combined with riluzole, neuro-rehabilitation, and 6 weeks of lithium. Her ALSFRS-R score increased from 29 to 32, and FIM score increased from 48 to 64. The highlight of this case is halting of disease progression with symptomatic improvements over a period of 12 months after intervention (**Table 3** and **Figure 7**).

A 63-year-old man who underwent autologous intrathecal BMMNC transplantation as a therapy in a clinical case of MND followed by multidisciplinary neurorehabilitation showed improvements in muscle strength, fine motor activities, fasciculation, cramps, and walking (**Table 4**). ALSFRS-R score improved from 33 to 37; Berg's balance score improved from 43 to 50, and 6-minute walk test improved from 283.8 to 303.6 m. His FIM score remained unchanged at 113. These improvements may be attributed to cellular therapy along with standard treatment and neurorehabilitation [99].

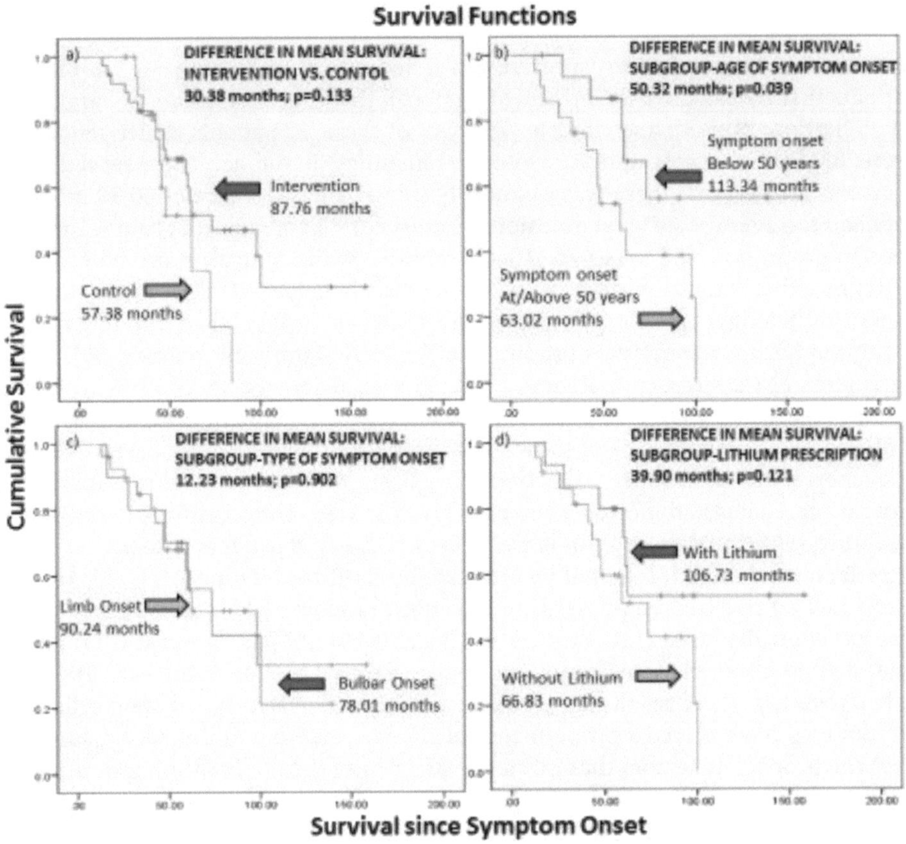

Figure 5.
(a) Kaplan-Meier survival analysis comparing the mean survival duration of the intervention (n = 37) and control group (n = 20) from Sharma et al. [16]. Mean survival duration of patients in the intervention group was higher than the control group by a clinically significant difference of 30.38 months. (b) Subgroup analysis of the effect of age of symptom onset on survival duration within the intervention group, from Sharma et al. [16] shows significantly higher survival of those with an onset of symptoms above 50 years of age (p = 0.039).
(c) Subgroup analysis of the effect of the type of symptom onset (limb vs. bulbar) on survival duration in the intervention group shows higher survival of patients with limb onset of symptoms by 12.23 months.
(d) Subgroup analysis of the effect of lithium prescription on survival duration within the intervention group shows a clinically higher survival of 106.73 months of the group prescribed with lithium. This is a clinically significant difference of 30.90 months as compared to controls, whose average survival was 66.83 months.

Prognostic factor		Median survival since symptom onset	*p*-Value
Lithium	Given	106.73 (15.69)	0.121
	Not given	66.83 (7.52)	
Age at symptom onset	Below 50 years	113.34 (15.45)	0.039*
	Above 50 years	63.02 (7.7)	
Type of symptom onset	Limb	78.01 (14.23)	0.902
	Bulbar	90.24 (13.27)	

*Statistically significant ($p < 0.05$).

Table 1.
Summary of prognostic factors affecting patient survival in the intervention group, from Sharma et al. [16]. Standard deviation is indicated in parentheses.

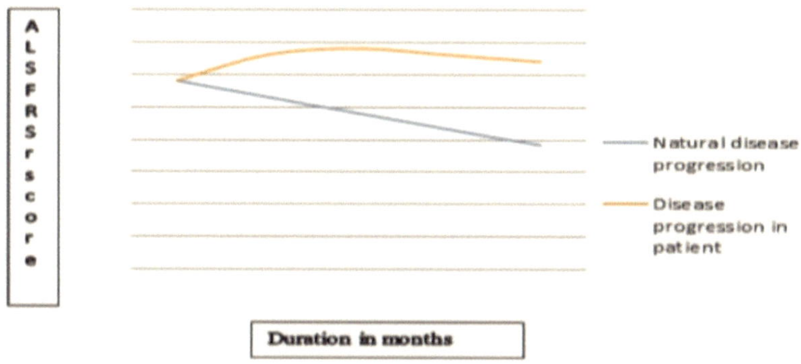

Figure 6.
Maintenance of a 40-year-old female ALS patient's condition over the period of 17 months. Disease progression in patient (red) was compared using ALSFRS-R with average values obtained from de Carvalho et al. (blue) at 0, 5, 15, and 17 months [97].

Outcome measures	At assessment before the first transplant	At 5 months after the first transplant (just before the second transplant)	At 15 months after the first transplant	At 17 months after the first transplant
ALSFRS-R	36	36	36	33
FIM	113	113	113	113

Table 2.
ALSFRS-R and FIM instrument scores of the patient remain stable as compared to assessment, when followed up at 5, 15, and 17 months.

Outcome measures	At assessment before the first transplant	At 2 months after the first transplant	At 6 months after the first transplant	At 9 months after the first transplant	At 12 months after the first transplant
ALSFRS-R	29	33	34	33	32
FIM	48	72	73	71	64

Table 3.
ALSFRS-R and FIM scores of a 41-year-old female ALS patient measured at assessment and after intervention (at 2, 6, 9, and 12 months post autologous BMMNC transplantation) depict stark improvement.

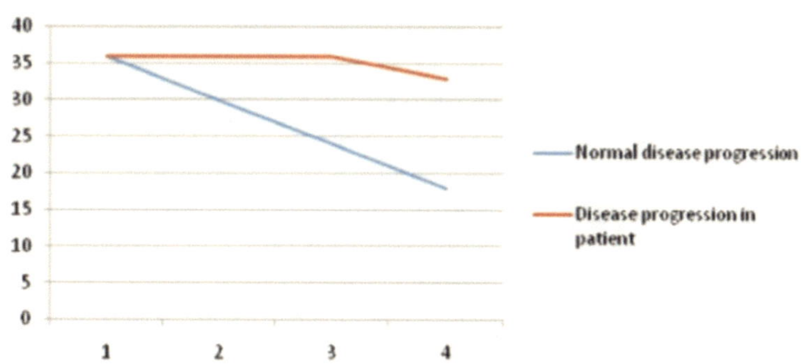

Figure 7.
ALSFRS-R and FIM scores were marked at 2, 4, 6, 9, and 12 months for this patient. ALSFRS-R score was measured across survival duration (in months) to compare the disease progression of this patient with natural disease progression in ALS, as measured by de Carvalho et al. [97]. The patient's condition was maintained over a period of 12 months.

Outcome measures	Pre-first SCT	At 6 months post the first SCT
ALSFRS-R	33	37
FIM	113	113
6-minute walk test	283.8 m	303.6 m
Berg's balance score	43	50

Table 4.
Improvements in outcome measures over a period of 6 months in a 63-year-old male ALS patient. ALSFRS-R, FIM, and 6-minute walk test were measured. Although not standard, Berg's balance test was administered to assess his balance.

A 29-year-old female patient with anterior horn cell involvement suffering from MND for 5 years presented with complaints of sudden onset of weakness in bilateral lower limbs post pregnancy. Her progressive condition was followed by gradual involvement of upper limbs also; EMG studies were also suggestive of MND. Her features were suggestive of pure motor system involvement affecting lower motor neurons. Post NRRT, she immediately showed clinical and functional improvements [17].

4.2.2.4 Unpublished data

4.2.2.4.1 Female hormones enhance the neuroprotective benefits of cellular transplantation in patients with amyotrophic lateral sclerosis (ALS)

The male/female ratio in ALS/MND worldwide points toward a lower incidence in females as compared to males. We hypothesized that this was due to a neuroprotective effect conferred by female hormones. In order to investigate this hypothesis, we designed a cohort study with 40 sequentially recruited ALS patients (28 males and 12 females) who were treated with stem cell therapy. To study the effect of reproductive hormones, patients were divided into pre- and postmenopausal women and men below and above 50 years of age.

We saw that percentage survival was highest in the premenopausal women (100%) followed by men below the age of 50 years (75%), postmenopausal women (60%), and men above the age of 50 years (45%). The disease progression was also slowest in the premenopausal women, followed by postmenopausal women, and men below 50 years of age; it was fastest in men above the age of 50 years (**Table 5**).

Group	Mean pre-ALSFRS-R	Mean post-ALSFRS-R	Difference	Average follow-up (months)	Percentage mortality
Premenopausal females (7)	26	23	3	20	0
Postmenopausal females (5)	21	14	7	14	40
Males below 50 years of age (16)	25	20	5	10	25
Males above 50 years of age (12)	32	25	7	13	55

Table 5.
Percentage mortalities across the four subgroups in a cohort study.

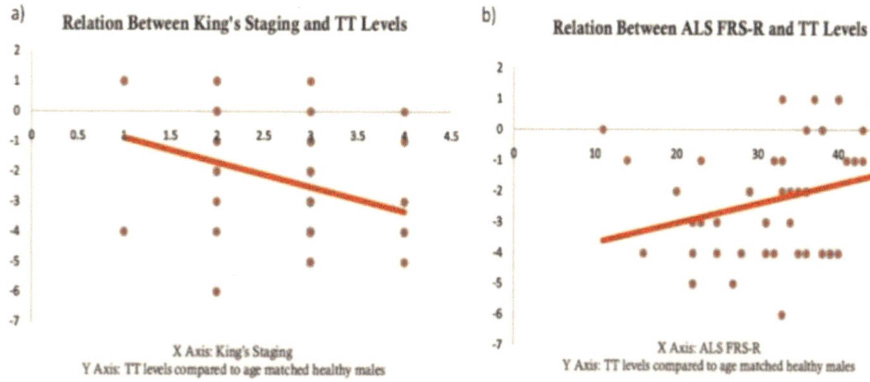

Figure 8.
Relationship of testosterone with (a) King's staging and (b) ALSFRS-R.

4.2.2.4.2 Correlation of testosterone levels with progression of amyotrophic lateral sclerosis: a cross-sectional study

We conducted an open-label nonrandomized cross-sectional study to interrogate the relationship of testosterone (TT) with disease progression. We found that 39 of the total 50 (78%) ALS patients had plasma TT levels lower than the mean levels in healthy, age-matched control males. We also found a decline in TT levels as the disease progressed on King's staging as well as ALSFRS-R (**Figure 8**). There was a statistically significant moderate monotonic correlation between ALSFRS-R scores and King's staging of patients with plasma testosterone levels (ALSFRS-R: r = +0.33;

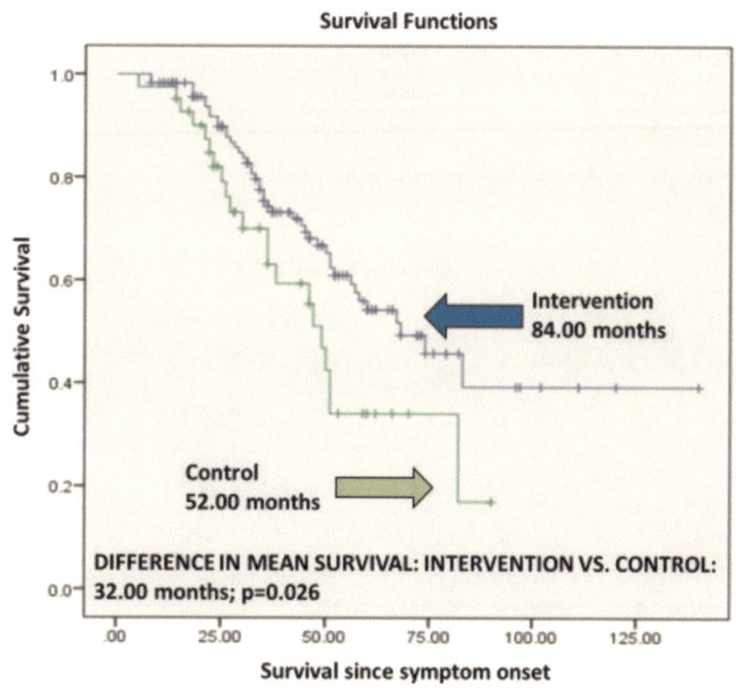

Figure 9.
Kaplan-Meier survival curves for control vs. intervention groups in our open-label study with a total of 157 subjects (intervention = 116; control = 41). On an average, the treated group survived for 32 months longer than the control group (p = 0.026).

King's staging: $r = -0.35$; $p = 0.01$). Taken together, these results suggest that reduced testosterone may exacerbate motor neuron loss or cause other etiopathological dysfunctions that remain to be elucidated.

4.2.2.4.3 Effect of intrathecal application of autologous bone marrow mononuclear cells on survival duration in ALS

We performed a large, open-label cohort study, which included 157 patients diagnosed with ALS from September 2013 to May 2017. About 116 patients who received cell transplantation (autologous BMMNCs) together with standard treatment formed the treatment group, and 41 patients who received only the standard treatment formed the control group (**Figure 9** and **Table 6**). We observed that on an average, the treated group survived for 32 months longer than the control group ($p = 0.026$).

Collectively, these findings were indicative of possible neuroprotective benefits of female reproductive hormones. Prognostic factors that predict improved survival and retarded disease progression include lithium co-administration, limb onset of symptoms, younger age of symptom onset, and, most importantly, presence of female hormones (**Figure 10**).

Characteristics			Intervention	Control
Total number of patients		157	116	41
Gender	Males	81	30	
	Females	35	11	
Mean age at symptom onset (years)		51 ± 11	53 ± 9	
Type of symptom onset	Bulbar	26	6	
	Limb	90	21	

Table 6.
Demographic data for an open-label study with 157 participants.

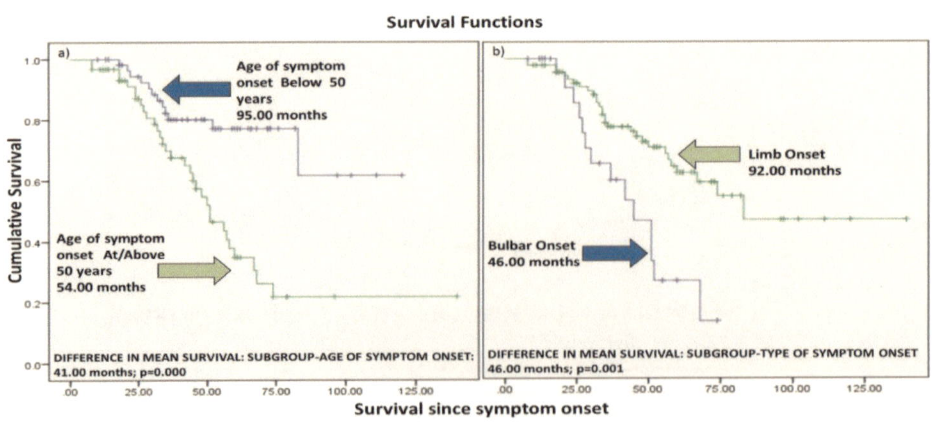

Figure 10.
(a) Subgroup analysis: survival duration was 46 months more in patients with limb onset as compared to bulbar onset ($p = 0.001$). Bulbar onset $n = 26$ patients and limb onset $n = 90$. (b) Survival duration was 41 months more in patients with age of symptom onset <50 years as compared to symptom onset at/above 50 years ($p < 0.000$).

5. Conclusion and future directions

Stem cell therapy is a novel, promising modality for the treatment of ALS/MND. Robust safety profiles, low risk-to-benefit ratio, and ease of access make this approach a strong contender in the race against ALS/MND. Consistently, autologous BMMNC therapy has been proven to mitigate disease progression; however, this response may be dependent on various factors, like age of symptom onset, gender, hormones, type of onset (limb vs. bulbar), and genetic makeup of the patient, to name a few. Younger patients—especially premenopausal females—may respond better to autologous BMMNC therapy. Stem cells combat tissue degeneration via a host of somatic and paracrine mechanisms, including neurogenesis, astrogliogenesis, neoangiogenesis, and immunomodulation. Multidisciplinary neurorehabilitation enhances the response to cellular therapy.

Although not a cure yet, a combinatorial approach integrating stem cell therapy, intensive neurorehabilitation, and current pharmacotherapeutic agents (e.g., riluzole, lithium, etc.) may be the best way forward. Studies that interrogate the genetics of patients and their family are the need of the hour, to enhance response to treatment and develop diagnostics and biomarkers. Also, the role of reproductive hormones such as progesterone, estradiol, and testosterone needs to be further explored. Larger clinical studies with stringent criteria are required to understand the efficacy of these combined methods in the treatment of ALS/MND. The current scenario suggests that autologous stem cell therapy can be considered along with standard treatment in carefully selected patients of ALS/MND.

Conflict of interest

The authors declare no conflict of interest in the writing of this chapter.

Appendix

See **Table 7**.

Authors, year, country (type of study, sample size)	Type of cells used (route of administration)	Results
Mazzini et al. [81], Italy (clinical trial, 7)	Autologous mesenchymal stem cells (intraspinal)	Slowing down of the linear decline of muscular strength was evident in four patients and improvement in strength in two patients in proximal lower limb muscles was observed
Deda et al. [18], Turkey (clinical trial, 13)	Bone marrow-derived hematopoietic progenitor stem cells (intraspinal)	9/13 (69.23%) patients improved as compared with their preoperative status, as confirmed by EMG
Martinez et al. [82], Mexico (controlled clinical trial, 10)	Autologous peripheral blood stem (intracerebral)	The survival of treated patients was statistically higher (p = 0.01) than untreated control patients
Prabhakar et al. [83], India (clinical trial—pilot study, 10)	Autologous bone marrow stem cells (intrathecal)	There was no significant deterioration in ALSFRS-R composite score from baseline at a 1-year follow-up (p = 0.090). The median survival post procedure was 18.0 months and median time to 4-point deterioration was 16.7 months

Authors, year, country (type of study, sample size)	Type of cells used (route of administration)	Results
Karussis et al. [31], Israel (phase I/phase II clinical trial, 19)	Autologous mesenchymal stem cells (intrathecal and intravenous)	The mean ALSFRS-R score remained stable during the first 6 months of observation. In ~80% of the patients, FVC values remained stable or above 70% for a time of 9 months and remained in ~60% of patients at 12 months after application. Signs of disease stabilization in some patients during the first 6 months after the intervention
Gamez et al. [84], Spain (observational study, 12)	Olfactory ensheathing cells (intracerebral) and autologous mesenchymal stromal cells (intrathecal + intravenous or only intrathecal)	No changes in the decline of FVC and ALSFRS-R compared with the disease's natural history were observed
Riley et al. [85], USA (phase I safety trial, 12)	Neural stem cells derived from a fetal spinal cord (intrathecal)	Procedural safety of unilateral and bilateral intraspinal lumbar microinjections has been suggested by the results of this trial
Petrou et al. [86], Israel (open-label proof-of-concept study, phase I/phase II and IIa)	Mesenchymal stem cells induced to secrete neurotrophic factors (intramuscular (IM), intrathecal (IT) or (IT+IM))	Progression rate of the ALSFRS-R score in the IT (or IT+IM)-treated patients was reduced from −1.2 to 0.6 ALSFRS-R points/month ($p = 0.052$), and the progression rate of the forced vital capacity reduced from −5.1% to −1.2%/month during the 6 months follow-up vs. pretreatment period
Blanquer et al. [34], Spain (clinical trial, pilot safety study, 11)	Autologous bone marrow stem cells (intraspinal)	7/11 (63.63%) patients remained stable post procedure
Mazzini et al. [21], Italy (clinical trial, long-term safety study, 9)	Autologous mesenchymal stem cells (intraspinal)	Brain MRI revealed no structural changes relative to baseline throughout follow-up. No deterioration noted in the psychosocial status as well
Huang et al. [19], China (controlled pilot study, 35)	Fetal olfactory ensheathing cells (intracerebral)	7/14 improved; 2/14 remained stable compared to the entry in the treated group, while only 1/17 of the patients remained stable within control
Glass et al. [22], USA (phase I clinical trial, 12)	Fetal neural stem cells (intraspinal)	Patients remained stable and tolerated the therapy well, as seen in clinical assessments at 6–18 months
Riley et al. [87], USA (phase I trial, 15)	NSI-566RSC-a human neural stem cell (intrathecal)	Cellular delivery to the cervical or thoracolumbar spinal cord was well tolerated by the patients
Sharma et al. [16], India (retrospective controlled cohort study, 57)	Autologous bone marrow mononuclear cells (intrathecal)	Mean survival duration of intervention was 87.76 months, which was higher than the control (57.38 months) or previous epidemiological studies. Survival duration was significantly ($p = 0.039$) higher in people with

Authors, year, country (type of study, sample size)	Type of cells used (route of administration)	Results
		the onset of the disease below 50 years of age. Limb onset and lithium also showed positive influence on the survival duration
Oh et al. [35], South Korea (single open-label phase I clinical trial, 8)	Mesenchymal stem cells (intrathecal)	Decline in the ALSFRS-R score was slow during the 6-month follow-up period
Rushkevich et al. [88], Belarus (controlled clinical trial, 10)	Autologous mesenchymal stem cells (intravenous, intrathecal)	Evaluation of the 12-month follow-up revealed slowing down of the disease progression in 10 patients
Ruiz-López et al. [89], Spain (phase I clinical trial, 11)	Autologous bone marrow stem cells (intramedullary)	All 11 patients were 100% stable
Syková et al. [36], Czech Republic (phase I/phase IIa prospective, nonrandomized, open-label clinical trial, 26)	Autologous mesenchymal stem cells (intrathecal)	A significant reduction/stabilization was found in ALSFRS-R decline at 3, 6, 9, and 12 months after treatment

All studies demonstrate safety of stem cells, except Glass et al. [22]. Safety in this table does not describe events unrelated to stem cell therapy.

Table 7.
Significant clinical studies employing stem cell therapy for treatment of ALS/MND, primarily from March 2009 to February 2019.

Author details

Alok Sharma[1], Hemangi Sane[2], Nandini Gokulchandran[3], Prerna Badhe[4], Amruta Paranjape[2,5]*, Radhika Pradhan[2], Rohit Das[5] and Hema Biju[5]

1 NeuroGen Brain and Spine Institute, Navi Mumbai, India

2 Department of Research and Development, NeuroGen Brain and Spine Institute, Navi Mumbai, India

3 Department of Medical Services and Clinical Research, NeuroGen Brain and Spine Institute, Navi Mumbai, India

4 Department of Regenerative Laboratory Services, NeuroGen Brain and Spine Institute, Navi Mumbai, India

5 Department of Neurorehabilitation, NeuroGen Brain and Spine Institute, Navi Mumbai, India

*Address all correspondence to: publications@neurogen.in

References

[1] Talbot K. Motor neuron disease: The bare essentials. Practical Neurology. 2009;**9**(5):303-309

[2] McDermott CJ, Shaw PJ. Diagnosis and management of motor neurone disease. BMJ. 2008;**336**(7645):658-662

[3] Marin B, Boumédiene F, Logroscino G, Couratier P, Babron M-C, Leutenegger AL, et al. Variation in worldwide incidence of amyotrophic lateral sclerosis: A meta-analysis. International Journal of Epidemiology. 2017;**46**(1):57-74

[4] Manjaly ZR, Scott KM, Abhinav K, Wijesekera L, Ganesalingam J, Goldstein LH, et al. The sex ratio in amyotrophic lateral sclerosis: A population based study. Amyotrophic Lateral Sclerosis: Official Publication of the World Federation of Neurology Research Group on Motor Neuron Diseases. 2010;**11**(5):439-442

[5] Mitchell JD, Callagher P, Gardham J, Mitchell C, Dixon M, Addison-Jones R, et al. Timelines in the diagnostic evaluation of people with suspected amyotrophic lateral sclerosis (ALS)/ motor neuron disease (MND)—A 20-year review: Can we do better? Amyotrophic Lateral Sclerosis: Official Publication of the World Federation of Neurology Research Group on Motor Neuron Diseases. 2010;**11**(6):537-541

[6] Jenkins TM, Hollinger H, McDermott CJ. The evidence for symptomatic treatments in amyotrophic lateral sclerosis. Current Opinion in Neurology. Oct 2014;**27**(5):524-531

[7] Miller RG, Mitchell JD, Lyon M, Moore DH. Riluzole for amyotrophic lateral sclerosis (ALS)/motor neuron disease (MND). Cochrane Database of Systematic Reviews. 2002;**2**:CD001447

[8] Ikeda K, Iwasaki Y. Edaravone, a free radical scavenger, delayed symptomatic and pathological progression of motor neuron disease in the wobbler mouse. PLoS ONE. 2015;**10**(10):e0140316

[9] Cruz MP. Nuedexta for the treatment of pseudobulbar affect. Pharmacology and Therapeutics. 2013;**38**(6):325-328

[10] Hardiman O. Multidisciplinary care in ALS: Expanding the team. Amyotrophic Lateral Sclerosis. 2012; **13**(2):165-165

[11] O'Brien M, Whitehead JB, Douglas Mitchell J. Multidisciplinary team working in motor neurone disease: Patient and family carer views. British Journal of Neuroscience Nursing. 2011; 7(4):580-585

[12] Paganoni S, Karam C, Joyce N, Bedlack R, Carter GT. Comprehensive rehabilitative care across the spectrum of amyotrophic lateral sclerosis. NeuroRehabilitation. 2015;**37**(1):53-68

[13] Sharma A, Gokulchandran N, Sane H, Nagrajan A, Paranjape A, Kulkarni P, et al. Autologous bone marrow mononuclear cell therapy for autism: An open label proof of concept study. Stem Cells International. 2013;**2013**:623875

[14] Chahine NA, Wehbe T, Rashed J, Hilal R, Elias N. Autologous bone marrow derived stem cells for the treatment of multiple sclerosis. International Journal of Stem Cells. 2016;**9**(2):207-212

[15] Sharma A, Sane H, Badhe P, Gokulchandran N, Kulkarni P, Lohiya M, et al. A clinical study shows safety and efficacy of autologous bone marrow mononuclear cell therapy to improve quality of life in muscular dystrophy patients. Cell Transplantation. 2013;**22** (1_suppl):127-138

[16] Sharma AK, Sane HM, Paranjape AA, Gokulchandran N, Nagrajan A,

D'sa M, et al. The effect of autologous bone marrow mononuclear cell transplantation on the survival duration in amyotrophic lateral sclerosis—A retrospective controlled study. American Journal of Stem Cells. 2015;**4**(1):50-65

[17] Sharma A, Badhe P, Shetty O, Vijaygopal P, Gokulchandran N, Jacob VC, et al. Autologous bone marrow derived stem cells for motor neuron disease with anterior horn cell involvement. The Bombay Hospital Journal. 2011;**53**(1):71-75

[18] Deda H, Inci MC, Kürekçi AE, Sav A, Kayihan K, Ozgün E, et al. Treatment of amyotrophic lateral sclerosis patients by autologous bone marrow-derived hematopoietic stem cell transplantation: A 1-year follow-up. Cytotherapy. 2009; **11**(1):18-25

[19] Huang H, Chen L, Xi H, Wang H, Zhang J, Zhang F, et al. Fetal olfactory ensheathing cells transplantation in amyotrophic lateral sclerosis patients: A controlled pilot study. Clinical Transplantation. 2008;**22**(6):710-718

[20] Mazzini L, Gelati M, Profico DC, Sgaravizzi G, Projetti Pensi M, Muzi G, et al. Human neural stem cell transplantation in ALS: Initial results from a phase I trial. Journal of Translational Medicine. 2015;**13**:17

[21] Mazzini L, Mareschi K, Ferrero I, Miglioretti M, Stecco A, Servo S, et al. Mesenchymal stromal cell transplantation in amyotrophic lateral sclerosis: A long-term safety study. Cytotherapy. 2012;**14**(1):56-60

[22] Glass JD, Boulis NM, Johe K, Rutkove SB, Federici T, Polak M, et al. Lumbar intraspinal injection of neural stem cells in patients with amyotrophic lateral sclerosis: Results of a phase I trial in 12 patients. Stem cells (Dayton, Ohio). 2012;**30**(6):1144-1151

[23] Stem Cell Basics II. stemcells.nih. gov [Internet]. Available from: https:// stemcells.nih.gov/info/basics/2.htm [Accessed: 16 October 2018]

[24] Marędziak M, Śmieszek A, Chrząstek K, Basinska K, Marycz K. Physical activity increases the total number of bone-marrow-derived mesenchymal stem cells, enhances their osteogenic potential, and inhibits their adipogenic properties. Stem Cells International. 2015;**2015**:11. Article ID: 379093

[25] Weissman IL. Stem cells: Units of development, units of regeneration, and units in evolution. Cell. 2000;**100**(1): 157-168

[26] Morrison SJ, Spradling AC. Stem cells and niches: Mechanisms that promote stem cell maintenance throughout life. Cell. 2008;**132**(4): 598-611

[27] Khademhosseini A, Karp JM, Gerecht-Nir S, Ferreira L, Annabi N, Sirabella D, et al. Chapter 32—Embryonic stem cells as a cell source for tissue engineering. In: Lanza R, Langer R, Vacanti J, editors. Principles of Tissue Engineering. 4th ed. Boston: Academic Press; 2014. pp. 609-638. Available from: http://www.sciencedirect.com/science/article/pii/B978012398358900032X [cited 8 October 2018]

[28] Stem Cell Basics V. stemcells.nih. gov [Internet]. Available from: https:// stemcells.nih.gov/info/basics/5.htm [Accessed: 16 October 2018]

[29] Gage FH. Mammalian neural stem cells. Science. 2000;**287**(5457): 1433-1438

[30] O'Donoghue K, Fisk NM. Fetal stem cells. Best Practice & Research. Clinical Obstetrics & Gynaecology. 2004;**18**(6): 853-875

[31] Karussis D, Karageorgiou C, Vaknin-Dembinsky A, Gowda-Kurkalli B, Gomori JM, Kassis I, et al. Safety and

immunological effects of mesenchymal stem cell transplantation in patients with multiple sclerosis and amyotrophic lateral sclerosis. Archives of Neurology. 2010;**67**(10):1187-1194

[32] Thurairajah K, Broadhead M, Balogh Z, Thurairajah K, Broadhead ML, Balogh ZJ. Trauma and stem cells: Biology and potential therapeutic implications. International Journal of Molecular Sciences. 2017;**18**(3):577

[33] Nagpal A, Choy FC, Howell S, Hillier S, Chan F, Hamilton-Bruce MA, et al. Safety and effectiveness of stem cell therapies in early-phase clinical trials in stroke: A systematic review and meta-analysis. Stem Cell Research & Therapy. Aug 30 2017;**8**(1):191

[34] Blanquer M, Moraleda JM, Iniesta F, Gómez-Espuch J, Meca-Lallana J, Villaverde R, et al. Neurotrophic bone marrow cellular nests prevent spinal motoneuron degeneration in amyotrophic lateral sclerosis patients: A pilot safety study. Stem cells (Dayton, Ohio). 2012;**30**(6):1277-1285

[35] Oh K-W, Moon C, Kim HY, Oh S-I, Park J, Lee JH, et al. Phase I trial of repeated intrathecal autologous bone marrow-derived mesenchymal stromal cells in amyotrophic lateral sclerosis. Stem Cells Translational Medicine. 2015; **4**(6):590-597

[36] Syková E, Rychmach P, Drahorádová I, Konrádová Š, Růžičková K, Voříšek I, et al. Transplantation of mesenchymal stromal cells in patients with amyotrophic lateral sclerosis: Results of phase I/IIa clinical trial. Cell Transplantation. 2017;**26**(4):647-658

[37] Waller-Wise R. Umbilical cord blood: Information for childbirth educators. The Journal of Perinatal Education. 2011;**20**(1):54-60

[38] Beane OS, Fonseca VC, Cooper LL, Koren G, Darling EM. Impact of aging on the regenerative properties of bone marrow-, muscle-, and adipose-derived mesenchymal stem/stromal cells. PLoS ONE. 2014;**9**(12):e115963

[39] Zuk PA, Zhu M, Mizuno H, Huang J, Futrell JW, Katz AJ, et al. Multilineage cells from human adipose tissue: Implications for cell-based therapies. Tissue Engineering. 2001;7(2):211-228

[40] Lin G, Garcia M, Ning H, Banie L, Guo Y-L, Lue TF, et al. Defining stem and progenitor cells within adipose tissue. Stem Cells and Development. 2008;**17**(6):1053-1063

[41] Takahashi K, Yamanaka S. Induction of pluripotent stem cells from mouse embryonic and adult fibroblast cultures by defined factors. Cell. 2006; **126**(4):663-676

[42] de Souza FT, de Souza FC, Mencalha AL. Human induced pluripotent stem cells from basic research to potential clinical applications in cancer. BioMed Research International. 2013;**2013**:11 (Article ID 430290)

[43] Blasco H, Mavel S, Corcia P, Gordon PH. The glutamate hypothesis in ALS: Pathophysiology and drug development. Current Medicinal Chemistry. 2014; **21**(31):3551-3575

[44] Glass CK, Saijo K, Winner B, Marchetto MC, Gage FH. Mechanisms underlying inflammation in neurodegeneration. Cell. 2010;**140**(6): 918-934

[45] Knott AB, Bossy-Wetzel E. Nitric oxide in health and disease of the nervous system. Antioxidants & Redox Signaling. 2009;**11**(3):541-553

[46] Smith EF, Shaw PJ, De Vos KJ. The role of mitochondria in amyotrophic lateral sclerosis. Neuroscience Letters. Jun 30 2017;**pii**: S0304-3940(17)30544-X

[47] Armon C. From snow to hill to ALS: An epidemiological odyssey in search of ALS causation. Journal of the Neurological Sciences. 2018;**391**:134-140

[48] Al-Chalabi A, Hardiman O. The epidemiology of ALS: A conspiracy of genes, environment and time. Nature Reviews. Neurology. 2013;**9**(11):617-628

[49] Pokrishevsky E, Grad LI, Yousefi M, Wang J, Mackenzie IR, Cashman NR. Aberrant localization of FUS and TDP43 is associated with misfolding of SOD1 in amyotrophic lateral sclerosis. PLoS ONE. 2012;**7**(4):e35050

[50] Keller BA, Volkening K, Droppelmann CA, Ang LC, Rademakers R, Strong MJ. Co-aggregation of RNA binding proteins in ALS spinal motor neurons: Evidence of a common pathogenic mechanism. Acta neuropathologica. 2012;**124**(5):733-747

[51] Maruyama H, Morino H, Ito H, Izumi Y, Kato H, Watanabe Y, et al. Mutations of optineurin in amyotrophic lateral sclerosis. Nature. 2010; **465**(7295):223-226

[52] Phruksaniyom C, Dharmasaroja P, Issaragrisil S. Bone marrow non-mesenchymal mononuclear cells induce functional differentiation of neuroblastoma cells. Experimental Hematology & Oncology. 2013;**2**:9

[53] Bhasin A, Srivastava MVP, Mohanty S, Vivekanandhan S, Sharma S, Kumaran S, et al. Paracrine mechanisms of intravenous bone marrow-derived mononuclear stem cells in chronic ischemic stroke. Cerebrovascular Diseases EXTRA. 2016;**6**(3):107-119

[54] Pastor D, Viso-León MC, Jones J, Jaramillo-Merchán J, Toledo-Aral JJ, Moraleda JM, et al. Comparative effects between bone marrow and mesenchymal stem cell transplantation in GDNF expression and motor function recovery in a motor neuron degenerative mouse model. Stem Cell Reviews. 2012;**8**(2):445-458

[55] Kamihata H, Matsubara H, Nishiue T, Fujiyama S, Tsutsumi Y, Ozono R, et al. Implantation of bone marrow mononuclear cells into ischemic myocardium enhances collateral perfusion and regional function via side supply of angioblasts, angiogenic ligands, and cytokines. Circulation. 2001;**104**(9):1046-1052

[56] Kim SH, Oh K-W, Jin HK, Bae J-S. Immune inflammatory modulation as a potential therapeutic strategy of stem cell therapy for ALS and neurodegenerative diseases. BMB Reports. 2018;**51**(11):545-546

[57] Gu R, Hou X, Pang R, Li L, Chen F, Geng J, et al. Human adipose-derived stem cells enhance the glutamate uptake function of GLT1 in SOD1(G93A)-bearing astrocytes. Biochemical and Biophysical Research Communications. 2010;**393**(3):481-486

[58] Mezey É, Chandross KJ, Harta G, Maki RA, McKercher SR. Turning blood into brain: Cells bearing neuronal antigens generated in vivo from bone marrow. Science. 2000;**290**(5497): 1779-1782

[59] Sasaki M, Honmou O, Akiyama Y, Uede T, Hashi K, Kocsis J. Transplantation of an acutely isolated bone marrow fraction repairs demyelinated adult rat spinal cord axons. GLIA. 2001;**35**(1):26-34

[60] Eglitis MA, Mezey É. Hematopoietic cells differentiate into both microglia and macroglia in the brains of adult mice. Proceedings of the National Academy of Sciences of the United States of America. 1997;**94**(8):4080-4085

[61] Wislet-Gendebien S, Bruyère F, Hans G, Leprince P, Moonen G, Rogister B. Nestin-positive mesenchymal stem cells favour the astroglial lineage in

neural progenitors and stem cells by releasing active BMP4. BMC Neuroscience. 2004;**5**:33

[62] Xu L, Yan J, Chen D, Welsh AM, Hazel T, Johe K, et al. Human neural stem cell grafts ameliorate motor neuron disease in SOD-1 transgenic rats. Transplantation. 2006;**82**(7):865

[63] López-González R, Kunckles P, Velasco I. Transient recovery in a rat model of familial amyotrophic lateral sclerosis after transplantation of motor neurons derived from mouse embryonic stem cells. Cell Transplantation. 2009;**18** (10–11):1171-1181

[64] Boucherie C, Schäfer S, Lavand'homme P, Maloteaux J-M, Hermans E. Chimerization of astroglial population in the lumbar spinal cord after mesenchymal stem cell transplantation prolongs survival in a rat model of amyotrophic lateral sclerosis. Journal of Neuroscience Research. 2009;**87**(9):2034-2046

[65] Kim H, Kim HY, Choi MR, Hwang S, Nam K-H, Kim H-C, et al. Dose-dependent efficacy of ALS-human mesenchymal stem cells transplantation into cisterna magna in SOD1-G93A ALS mice. Neuroscience Letters. 2010; **468**(3):190-194

[66] Xu L, Shen P, Hazel T, Johe K, Koliatsos VE. Dual transplantation of human neural stem cells into cervical and lumbar cord ameliorates motor neuron disease in SOD1 transgenic rats. Neuroscience Letters. 2011;**494**(3): 222-226

[67] Bigini P, Veglianese P, Andriolo G, Cova L, Grignaschi G, Caron I, et al. Intracerebroventricular administration of human umbilical cord blood cells delays disease progression in two murine models of motor neuron degeneration. Rejuvenation Research. 2011;**14**(6):623-639

[68] Wyatt TJ, Rossi SL, Siegenthaler MM, Frame J, Robles R, Nistor G, et al. Human motor neuron progenitor transplantation leads to endogenous neuronal sparing in 3 models of motor neuron loss. Stem Cells International. May 23 2011;**2011**(2011):207230

[69] Lee JC, Seong J, Kim SH, Lee SJ, Cho YJ, An J, et al. Replacement of microglial cells using clodronate liposome and bone marrow transplantation in the central nervous system of SOD1(G93A) transgenic mice as an in vivo model of amyotrophic lateral sclerosis. Biochemical and Biophysical Research Communications. 2012;**418**(2):359-365

[70] Uccelli A, Milanese M, Principato MC, Morando S, Bonifacino T, Vergani L, et al. Intravenous mesenchymal stem cells improve survival and motor function in experimental amyotrophic lateral sclerosis. Molecular medicine (Cambridge, Mass.). 2012;**18**: 794-804

[71] Garbuzova-Davis S, Rodrigues MCO, Mirtyl S, Turner S, Mitha S, Sodhi J, et al. Multiple intravenous administrations of human umbilical cord blood cells benefit in a mouse model of ALS. PLoS ONE. Feb 3 2012;**7** (2):e31254

[72] Hefferan MP, Galik J, Kakinohana O, Sekerkova G, Santucci C, Marsala S, et al. Human neural stem cell replacement therapy for amyotrophic lateral sclerosis by spinal transplantation. PLoS ONE. Aug 20 2012;**7**(8):e42614

[73] Popescu IR, Nicaise C, Liu S, Bisch G, Knippenberg S, Daubie V, et al. Neural progenitors derived from human induced pluripotent stem cells survive and differentiate upon transplantation into a rat model of amyotrophic lateral sclerosis. Stem Cells Translational Medicine. 2013;**2**(3):167-174

[74] Lee HJ, Kim KS, Ahn J, Bae HM, Lim I, Kim SU. Human motor neurons generated from neural stem cells delay clinical onset and prolong life in ALS mouse model. PLoS ONE. May 20 2014; **9**(5):e97518

[75] Sun H, Hou Z, Yang H, Meng M, Li P, Zou Q, et al. Multiple systemic transplantations of human amniotic mesenchymal stem cells exert therapeutic effects in an ALS mouse model. Cell and Tissue Research. 2014; **357**(3):571-582

[76] Kondo T, Funayama M, Tsukita K, Hotta A, Yasuda A, Nori S, et al. Focal transplantation of human iPSC-derived glial-rich neural progenitors improves lifespan of ALS mice. Stem Cell Reports. 2014;**3**(2):242-249

[77] Izrael M, Slutsky SG, Admoni T, Cohen L, Granit A, Hasson A, et al. Safety and efficacy of human embryonic stem cell-derived astrocytes following intrathecal transplantation in SOD1G93A and NSG animal models. Stem Cell Research & Therapy. 2018; **9**(1):152

[78] Thomsen GM, Avalos P, Ma AA, Alkaslasi M, Cho N, Wyss L, et al. Transplantation of neural progenitor cells expressing glial cell line-derived neurotrophic factor into the motor cortex as a strategy to treat amyotrophic lateral sclerosis. Stem Cells. 2018;**36**(7): 1122-1131

[79] Morrice JR, Gregory-Evans CY, Shaw CA. Animal models of amyotrophic lateral sclerosis: A comparison of model validity. Neural Regeneration Research. 2018;**13**:2050-4

[80] Moura MC, Novaes MRCG, Zago YSSP, Eduardo EJ, Casulari LA. Efficacy of stem cell therapy in amyotrophic lateral sclerosis: A systematic review and meta-analysis. Journal of Clinical Medical Research. 2016;**8**(4):317-324

[81] Mazzini L, Fagioli F, Boccaletti R, Mareschi K, Oliveri G, Olivieri C, et al. Stem cell therapy in amyotrophic lateral sclerosis: A methodological approach in humans. Amyotrophic Lateral Sclerosis: Official Publication of the World Federation of Neurology Research Group on Motor Neuron Diseases. 2003; **4**(3):158-161

[82] Martinez HR, Gonzalez-Garza MT, Moreno-Cuevas JE, Caro E, Gutierrez-Jimenez E, Segura JJ. Stem-cell transplantation into the frontal motor cortex in amyotrophic lateral sclerosis patients. Cytotherapy. 2009;**11**(1):26-34

[83] Prabhakar S, Marwaha N, Lal V, Sharma RR, Rajan R, Khandelwal N. Autologous bone marrow-derived stem cells in amyotrophic lateral sclerosis: A pilot study. Neurology India. 2012; **60**(5):465-469

[84] Gamez J, Carmona F, Raguer N, Ferrer-Sancho J, Martín-Henao GA, Martí-Beltrán S, et al. Cellular transplants in amyotrophic lateral sclerosis patients: An observational study. Cytotherapy. 2010;**12**(5):669-677

[85] Riley J, Federici T, Polak M, Kelly C, Glass J, Raore B, et al. Intraspinal stem cell transplantation in amyotrophic lateral sclerosis: A phase I safety trial, technical note, and lumbar safety outcomes. Neurosurgery. 2012;**71**(2): 405-416; discussion 416

[86] Petrou P, Gothelf Y, Argov Z, Gotkine M, Levy YS, Kassis I, et al. Safety and clinical effects of mesenchymal stem cells secreting neurotrophic factor transplantation in patients with amyotrophic lateral sclerosis: Results of phase 1/2 and 2a clinical trials. JAMA Neurology. 2016; **73**(3):337-344

[87] Riley J, Glass J, Feldman EL, Polak M, Bordeau J, Federici T, et al. Intraspinal stem cell transplantation in

amyotrophic lateral sclerosis: A phase I trial, cervical microinjection, and final surgical safety outcomes. Neurosurgery. 2014;**74**(1):77-87

[88] Rushkevich YN, Kosmacheva SM, Zabrodets GV, Ignatenko SI, Goncharova NV, Severin IN, et al. The use of autologous mesenchymal stem cells for cell therapy of patients with amyotrophic lateral sclerosis in Belarus. Bulletin of Experimental Biology and Medicine. 2015;**159**(4):576-581

[89] Ruiz-López FJ, Blanquer M. Autologous bone marrow mononuclear cells as neuroprotective treatment of amyotrophic lateral sclerosis. Neural Regeneration Research. 2016;**11**(4): 568-569

[90] Brooks BR, Miller RG, Swash M, Munsat TL, World Federation of Neurology Research Group on Motor Neuron Diseases. El Escorial revisited: Revised criteria for the diagnosis of amyotrophic lateral sclerosis. Amyotrophic Lateral Sclerosis: Official Publication of the World Federation of Neurology Research Group on Motor Neuron Diseases. 2000;**1**(5):293-299

[91] Yoon SH, Shim YS, Park YH, Chung JK, Nam JH, Kim MO, et al. Complete spinal cord injury treatment using autologous bone marrow cell transplantation and bone marrow stimulation with granulocyte macrophage-colony stimulating factor: Phase I/II clinical trial. Stem Cells. 2007; **25**(8):2066-2073

[92] Richman CM, Kinnealey A, Hoffman PC. Granulopoietic effects of lithium on human bone marrow in vitro. Experimental Hematology. 1981;**9**(4): 449-455

[93] Hashimoto R, Takei N, Shimazu K, Christ L, Lu B, Chuang D-M. Lithium induces brain-derived neurotrophic factor and activates TrkB in rodent cortical neurons: An essential step for neuroprotection against glutamate excitotoxicity. Neuropharmacology. 2002;**43**(7):1173-1179

[94] Fornai F, Longone P, Cafaro L, Kastsiuchenka O, Ferrucci M, Manca ML, et al. Lithium delays progression of amyotrophic lateral sclerosis. Proceedings of the National Academy of Sciences of the United States of America. 2008;**105**(6):2052-2057

[95] Morrison KE, Dhariwal S, Hornabrook R, Savage L, Burn DJ, Khoo TK, et al. Lithium in patients with amyotrophic lateral sclerosis (LiCALS): A phase 3 multicentre, randomised, double-blind, placebo-controlled trial. Lancet Neurology. 2013;**12**(4):339-345. DOI: 10.1016/S1474-4422(13)70037-1

[96] Verstraete E, Veldink JH, Huisman MHB, Draak T, Uijtendaal EV, van der Kooi AJ, et al. Lithium lacks effect on survival in amyotrophic lateral sclerosis: A phase IIb randomised sequential trial. Journal of Neurology, Neurosurgery, and Psychiatry. 2012;**83**(5):557-564

[97] de Carvalho M, Scotto M, Lopes A, Swash M. Quantitating progression in ALS. Neurology. 2005;**64**(10):1783-1785

[98] Sane H, Sharma A, Gokulchandran N, Kalburgi S, Paranjape A, Badhe P. Neurorestoration in amyotrophic lateral sclerosis—A case report. Journal of Stem cells and Regenerative Medicine. 2016; **2**(1):29-37

[99] Sharma A, Sane H, Paranjape A, Sawant D, Inamdar S, Gokulchandran N, et al. Cellular therapy in motor neuron disease: A case report. International Journal of Recent Advances in Multidisciplinary Research. 2017;**4**(5):2605-2609

Chapter 4

Introduction to Novel Motor Neuron Disease

Humberto Foyaca Sibat and Lourdes de Fátima Ibañez Valdés

Abstract

Motor neuron disease (MND) is a progressive and fatal neuromuscular disease; the most common and severe form of MND presentation is amyotrophic lateral sclerosis (ALS), commonly known as Lou Gehrig's disease. The majority of ALS patients die within 2–5 years of receiving a diagnosis. Familial ALS is a hereditary form of the disease and accounts for 5–10% of cases, whereas the remaining cases have no clearly defined etiology. ALS affects persons of all ethnicities and races; currently, no curative treatment for ALS is available worldwide. ALS is also the major adult-onset MND and is clinically, pathologically, and genetically associated with fronto-temporal dementia in some cases, which is the second cause of dementia in elderly people. However, MND does not affect sphincter, sexual function, or eye movements. MND is the most common degenerative disorder affecting the upper and lower motor neurons at the same time. Most of the patients presenting MND in our series complained of muscle weakness, muscle wasting, fasciculation, and spasticity plus lower cranial nerve disturbances. According to our bibliographic studies, apart from nusinersen, it seems to be that riluzole and edaravone also improve motor neuron function by acting on SK channels.

Keywords: motor neuron disease, amyotrophic lateral sclerosis, spinal muscular atrophy, riluzole, edaravone

1. Introduction

Motor neuron disease is composed of a group of rare neurodegenerative disorders, such as amyotrophic lateral sclerosis (ALS), spinal muscular atrophy (SMA), hereditary spastic paraplegia, primary lateral sclerosis, progressive muscular atrophy, pseudobulbar palsy, O'Sullivan-McLeod syndrome, and Madras motor neuron disease, which are fatal in 50% of affected people within 15–20 months after diagnosis. MND is a progressive neuromuscular disease with a fatal outcome; the commonest clinical presentation of MND presentation is ALS, commonly known as Lou Gehrig's disease. Most of ALS patients pass away within 2–5 years of confirmed a diagnosis. Familial ALS (ALSf) is a hereditary presentation of the disease and accounts for 5–10% of affected people. ALS affects persons of all ethnicities worldwide; no cure for ALS has yet been available at any country. Sometimes, ALS is clinically, pathologically, and genetically associated with fronto-temporal dementia, which is the second cause of dementia in elderly people. In our first book, we reviewed all previous chapters published by INTECH, and in the Introductory Chapter, readers could find summarized information about all publications on ALS made by INTECH. Trying to illustrate the reached progress, we displayed this information grouped by topics and countries in two graphics. As we saw on that book, the number of publications written about ALS increased remarkably for the past 4 years. To have some idea of this phenomenon, be informed that INTECH published more than 40 chapters on ALS in this period of time, and these books "Amyotrophic Lateral Sclerosis," "Current Advances on Amyotrophic Lateral Sclerosis," and others are fully available on line, for free. Therefore, why we are going to publish another chapter? All novel information about MND were not published. Therefore, some aspects published in 2012 need to be update because new ideas, proposals, findings, experiences, and many other's knowledge have been arising despite of this short period of time. Therefore, for the benefit of the readership community, we included update information not reported before, mainly new contribution of aberrant astrocytes to MND damage and death in the SOD1G93A rat experimental model of ALS; novel genetics studies on ALS; an update of the structural and functional consequences of the spinal muscular atrophy-linked mutations of the survival motor neuron protein; stem cell therapy for MND; and the novel treatment for SMA and ALS in the introductory chapter of this book. Compromises have been inevitable to accommodate our visual and factual updated information in a book of his characteristic on top of many chapters about the same issue published recently.

MND does not affect sphincter, sexual function, or eye movements [1]. Although ALS is not associated with thermoregulatory dysfunction, its progression can affect intensively important cerebral regions that control body temperature and affect multiple functions of this homeostatic activity. Nevertheless, experimental ALS animals can display altered thermoregulation as a consequence of affected energy homeostasis. Indirect evidence suggests, performing studies on the body temperature regulatory system, both as a possible modifier of disease progression in ALS and as a potential biomarker [2].

Although edaravone and riluzole do not cure MND/ALS, it seems to be that both medications can slow its progression. The prevalence of ALS in America was 5.2 per 100,000 populations with a total of 16,583 cases identified from January 1 to December 31, 2015 [3].

MND is the most common degenerative disorder, which affects the upper and lower motor neurons at the same time. There are different clinical modalities of MND being ALS the commonest one, and its incidence is around 1–3 patients every 100,000 people [4, 5].

The higher incidence of ALS is in patients with 60 and 70 years of age, but some younger cases (20–30 years of age) have been reported as well [4]. Between 5 and 10% of the patients have a familiar origin due to Mendelian autosomal dominant transmission.

Most of the patients presenting MND in our series complain of muscle weakness, muscle wasting, fasciculation, and spasticity plus cranial nerve disturbances from the lower brainstem.

The most frequent mutation seen in the familial form of ALS (ALSf) occurs on the gene of superoxide dismutase 1 (SOD1) and on the chromosome 9, among others. The decreased endovascular factor and the hereditary hemochromatosis protein are also genetic mutations. Some variations in the number of copies of Genes 1 and 2 that codify the motor neuron survival factors have been reported [6]. No correlation investigations have been done. However, some genome-wide studies in patients presenting ALS show a series of loci confirming a greater susceptibility to develop the disease such as kinase carbohydrate (FGGY), dipeptidyl-peptidase 6 (DPP6), and Type 2 inositol triphosphate receptor [7–9]. Most of these findings were not able to be replicated in further investigations done. At present, there is not specific cure for this deadly disorder as was mentioned before.

Long time ago, a nitrogenic expansion on the gene C9ORF72 was observed in a number of patients presenting ALS associated with Chromosome 9, which brought more clarity in the ethiopathogenesis of ALS [10, 11], but these findings are also seen in patients presenting fronto-temporal dementia (FTD) and ALS-FTD [10, 11]. Below, we will deliver more comments about this topic.

Future genetic investigations should be focused on non-European populations in order to bring more clarity on new pathogenic loci.

In the forthcoming years, the exome study that is an emerging field will bring novel information about some implicated genes in ALSf.

In 2018, Thompson et al. [12] used a high-throughput proteomic process to distinguish new biomarkers in patient's cerebrospinal fluid (CSF), and they found that three macrophage-derived chitinases had increased concentration in ALS: chitinase-3-like protein 1, chitotriosidase, and chitinase-3-like protein 2. Elevated CHI3L1 was commonly seen in ALS, while CHI3L2 and CHIT1 levels did not. Their results confirmed the important role of macrophage activity in pathogenesis of ALS.

Decreased cough capacity is almost always present in respiratory tract infection and is the most important cause of respiratory failure in ALS patients. Other authors determined whether the lung function measurement could identify the cough function in ALS patients with respiratory tract infection. After screening 48 patients presenting ALS, they found only four presenting a remarkable cough with no assistance. The data that identified unassisted cough effectiveness are peak cough flow. These investigators highlighted that the effectiveness of assisted and unassisted cough function depends on the peak cough flow reached [13].

It is well known that MND does not affect the motor neurons at the oculomotor nucleus in the midbrain. Because it could be remarkably advantageous if neurons of motor system resilience can be modeled in vitro, some authors reached elevated quantities of oculomotor neurons from embryonic stem cells in mouse through transient over expression of PHOX2A in nerve cell progenitors, and they confirmed, using immunocytochemistry techniques, electrophysiology studies, and RNA sequencing, that in vitro-generated neurons are bona fide oculomotor neuron cells based on their neuron properties and similarity to their counterpart in rodent (in vivo) and human beings [14].

Increased cortical excitability, thought to reflect pathological changes in the balance of local excitatory and inhibitory neuronal influences that are commonly seen in patients presenting ALS and non-invasive brain stimulation (NIBS), has been shown to modulate cortical activity, with some protocols showing effects that outlast the stimulation by months. Therefore, NIBS has been proposed as a probable candidate to approach therapeutically these disorders associated with pathological neurophysiology activity, such as ALS, among others [15].

ALS type 8 (ALS8) is a familial presentation of MND, with an important anterior horn cell degeneration, due to mutation of the vesicle-associated membrane protein-associated protein B. Some authors compare the cognitive function of patients with ALS8 and a control group composed by healthy people in order to screen behavioral features in ALS8 patients. These authors found that ALS8 patients showed minimal deficits in executive functions. The total amount of ALS8 patients and the control group have the same scores of facial emotion recognition. They also determined an important clinical expression of psychiatric disorder such as anxiety and depression in 36 and 27% of patients, respectively. However, behavioral disturbances were present in around 30% of participants. They concluded that these patients had mild executive problems and behavioral problems such as apathy, mood disorder, and stereotypic behavior, which suggest that ALS8 is not a motor disorder only, and it is associated with minor cognitive and behavioral changes [16].

Because one of the most effective clinical strategies for SMA is to protect the anterior horn cell, apart from nusinersen (that is a very expensive medication), one anti-epileptic medication levetiracetam has been used as well.

Kepra (levetiracetam) provoked neurite elongation in SMA-iPSCs-MNs. TUNEL-positive anterior horn cell was significantly decreased by kepra in SMA-iPSCs-MNs. On the other hand, the expression level of cleaved-caspase 3 was diminished by levetiracetam in SMA-iPSCs-MNs. Furthermore, kepra improved impaired mitochondrial function in SMA-iPSCs-MNs. On the other hand, kepra did not modify the expression level of SMN protein in SMA-iPSCs-MNs. These results suggest that kepra has a neuroprotective effect for SMA [17].

For patients presenting SMA (most common reason of inherited infant mortality), the gene therapy seems to be the most effective strategy [18].

Another therapeutic modality to treat ALS is the noninvasive brain stimulation (NIBS), which has been shown to modulate cortical activity, with some protocols leading effects that outlast the stimulation by months. NIBS have been suggested as a potential treatment choice in those processes with associated changes in the cortical neurophysiology [15].

A total of 25 genes associated with ALSf and ALS (sporadic form), mutations in fused-in-sarcoma (FUS) and superoxide dismutase 1 (SOD1) have been intensively studied in the past, focusing on modified excitability of motor neurons. Based on their personal experience, Peikkert et al. [19] proposed that the 4-aminopyridine (4-AP), which is a potassium channel blocker, can be utilized as a probable therapy *for ALS patients* due to its demonstrated hypo excitability and high frequency of apoptosis in a FUS/SOD1-ALS-induced multi-potent stem cell from selected motor neuron; they also found that this process is partly reversible by 4-AP.

One of the clinical presentations of MND is SMA, which encompasses a group of autosomal recessively inherited degenerative neuromuscular diseases. SMA is an inherited disorder that causes progressive lesions on the anterior horn cell leading to weakness or paralysis of the affected limbs, and it is caused by elimination or mutation of survival motor neuron (SMN) 1 gene. It is well known that homozygous damage and loss of functional mutations in the survival motor neuron 1 gene (SMN1) at the chromosome 5q13 are the main cause of SMA, which affect 1 in 11,000 newborn infants.

SMA usually has a very poor prognosis after rapidly progressive weakness and early mortality. However, a new medication named Nusinersen has been released for the treatment of all forms of SMA (not on mechanical ventilation) with very good results. In December 2016, this medication was approved in the United States. Nusinersen, an antisense oligonucleotide (ASO), is administered directly into CSF. It alters *SMN2* pre-RNA splicing, so exon 7 is included, increasing expression of functional SMN protein. *Efficacy assessments for patients receiving nusinersen are based on serial assessments of performance on age-appropriate standardized motor scales. Treatment requires complex financial and logistics because of the very high drug cost, intrathecal administration, and medical fragility of the patients. Treatment implementation also engenders ethical considerations related to cost, insurance coverage, limited clinical data on groups of patients not in clinical trials, and questions of duration of treatment* [20].

One in 50 asymptomatic people carries this autosomal recessive neuromuscular code causing SMA in one over 10,000 live births [21].

Based on age at onset, the highest milestone reached, and phenotypic severity: SMA has been separated into four different subgroups such as "Nonsitters" (Type I), "sitters" (Type II), "walkers" (Type III), and "adult onset" (Type IV) [22].

At the present moment, many patients got confirmation of diagnose very late, or the treatment is administered in advance stages. Therefore, poor response is often obtained.

Fortunately, some screening programs are available and accurately and then to identify children in pre-symptomatic stages is possible [23]. However, because some children develop their clinical manifestation far from birth then to decide when to initiate the treatment and whom qualify for therapy is a dilemma.

The majority of SMN2 pre-mRNA transcripts undergo alternative splicing due to a nucleotide substitution leading to exclusion of exon 7. Degradation of the resulting truncated SMN protein is very fast, and the overall lack of full-length SMN protein causes permanent damage on anterior horn cell of the spinal cord [23].

In patients with onset of the disease beyond six months of age, large phase 3 trials confirmed improvement in motor activities, very high event-free and remarkable survival in infantile-onset SMA3, also significant improvement in Expanded version of the Hammersmith Functional Motor Scale scores has been recorded [24, 25].

The copy number of the homologous SMN2 gene is inversely correlated with SMA severity and encoded by SMN1 (except for lack of exon 7), which is identical to the cDNA encoded by SMN2.

Currently, for the therapy of SMA, there are pipelines developed by antisense oligonucleotide (ASO), also available for Huntington disease, ALS, spinocerebellar ataxias, Parkinson disease, and Alzheimer disease, among other options, and the pharmaceutical industry on ASO development has been delivering a promising therapeutic approach. The key care concern to MND patients has been developed, and expert consensus guidelines delivered, and best management for lung diseases, nutritional problems, and palliative care has also been reached. However, in this chapter, we will discuss novel aspects related to treatment and other therapeutic procedures later on.

In pre-symptomatic SMA patient's Types I–III released interim results of a phase 2 trial evaluating the effects of Nusinersen have been done [23].

Some investigators have been working on stage of improvement after the treatment of SMA and confirmed that the first published data supported important good results on the motor function and quality of life from animal models with early restoration of SMN levels for those studied within the first 3 postnatal days. However, for those treated beyond 5 postnatal days, the level of recovery was low, while delivered treatment after 10 postnatal days, it showed no improvement and died [26].

One of the problems found in our preliminary review is the big number of SMA patients diagnosed at late stage. We found Type I patient with 4 months after onset and Type III with 10 months or more after onset [27, 28].

However, newborn screening programs have been a successful process for identifying affected children at an asymptomatic stage, leading to pre-symptomatic initiation of treatment before irreversible anterior horn cell lesion appears. To perform screening methods before birth are certain, and they available and willing to deliver the possibility of distinguish patients at the beginning of pregnancy, giving a chance to perform a prenatal therapeutic management.

Taiwan and Belgium, also have screening programs for SMA, but in America, the leader and an important number of states, further clinical trials have been implemented to evaluate the applicability and economic advantages. Unfortunately, around 5% of mutations in the SMN1 cannot de identified [23].

Chorionic villus sampling or amniocentesis to identify children with higher risk for SMA with an elevated percentage of accuracy can be done, if it is performed during the 10–14 or 15–20 weeks of pregnancy. These procedures can be dangerous for the mother and the baby to be done in *high-risk pregnancies with proven carrier status of the parents recommended* [23]. Nevertheless, isolating circulating fetal trophoblastic cells by noninvasive prenatal diagnosis techniques is also possible [29] or even getting from maternal blood cell-free fetal DNA [30]. These above-mentioned techniques allow to identify SMA in unborn children with 100% accuracy, promising a better future for SMA patients [23].

At this stage, it is also important to mention that significant ethical issues are involved in this genetic screening methodology and its need to be considered by the medical community before making these procedures fully available [31]. At the present moment, we are not quite sure how to predict disease severity accurately or even its presence because not all patients present clinical manifestation birth or because only few minimal sings are detectable. Treatment algorithm for SMA patients confirmed by newborn screening based on SMN1 deletion analysis in dried blood spots is available since 2005 [28]. Indications of treatment are based on the clinical phenotype of the patients and correlation of SMN2 copy numbers. All patients presenting 2–3 copies should be treated with the immediate effect according to NBS Multidisciplinary Working Group recommendations even if the child is asymptomatic with only one copy, but when four or more copies are present due to milder course of the disease, the treatment must be delayed [28].

In 2017, some authors studied a big number of SMA patients (n = 3500) trying to compare SMN2 copy number with their clinical information and found that patients with 1–4 copies have mild to severe phenotype, respectively, while there was an important overlap among patients with 2–3, confirming any possible phenotype [32], but more than 80% of patients in this group cohort carried two to three SMN2 copies, suggesting the similar problem in medical practice. In these cases, presenting two or three SMN2 copies to predict the severity of the disorder is not certain [23].

It is important to take into account that those SMA patients (families and siblings) presenting the same amount of SMN2 copies have another phenotype [33]; in the context, SMN1 (homozygous) mutations, SMN2 copies in people free of symptoms and signs, and even in SMA Type I have been found [34]. SMN2 transcripts and the SMN2 copy number do not show any correlation in a series of investigations done between 2001 and 2017 [35–38].

Following some recommendations delivered by the Phase 1 trial and studies on its pharmacological process, the investigators found that the half-life of nusinersen in the CFS is 163 days, and the ideal way for administration should be intrathecal (at the dosage of 12 mg) every 4 months. After that period of time, patients should receive five intrathecal injections within the first 6 months of treatment. These authors also confirmed that no correlation exits between concentrations of the CSF, age of the patients, and body weight [39, 40].

Based on results published by Luu et al., the doses of nusinersen according to the age of the patients produce more median exposures in the CSF, which suggest that prescribing fixed dosage programs through all age groups is the best choice [40]. For the other hand, Finkel et al. [41] conducted a Phase 2 dose-escalation investigation confirming that a single dose of 12 mg is better than 6 mg. The best way to assess the outcome for these patients is to measure the advantage of motor milestone, depending on ventilator machine, achievement of motor activities, clinical electrophysiological studies, and overall survival. Twenty patients younger than 1 year of age and less than 10 kg of body weight were screened, and these results confirmed the previous postulate [41]. The results from the small group studied in phase 2 clinical trials and the pharmacological studies done can accurately reflect clinical practice, is an interrogation still no responded.

Taking into account the great variability among SMA patients related to the age at disease onset, residual motor function, body weight, and fixed dose at the same intervals for patients, it seems to be remarkably inaccurate [23]. Reliable biomarkers and screening procedures for proper diagnosis at early stage of the disease are need more than ever if we are looking for longer survival and positive modifications of the patient outcome. If reliable biomarkers are not available, then determining the SMN protein level and epigenetic modifiers to provide confident information about the intensity of the process is mandatory. When more than three SMN2 copies are detectable, chance for life-saving treatment is not certain. In summary, novel screening techniques, procedures to predict the intensity of the disease, and reliable biomarkers, which support monitoring of the treatment, have been discovered and recently developed, but unfortunately, none of them provide an unequivocal explanation of the pathophysiology of SMA [23].

To develop more accurate diagnostic procedures including confident biomarkers, better therapeutic approaches, and novel predictors to determine the ideal dosing recommendation, more investigations are required. This is the only way to guarantee a reliable long-term treatment and successful outcome [23].

Two years ago, the European Medicines Agency finally approved nusinersen an antisense oligonucleotide (ASO) as the treatment of choice for SMA, and later, this medication has been considered as part of the treatment for patients with Type 2 SMA as well [23]. In patients with SMA presenting spinal bone deformities, severe contractures, scoliosis, spine fusion surgeries, and respiratory distress, the administration intrathecal of nusinersen could be a great challenge.

Recently, with the intention of assess, the accuracy, and feasibility of nusinersen administrated by lumbar puncture (LP) in young patients, Wurster et al. [42] studied in 93 patients in whom the LP is done, highlighting the amount of attempts performed, site of injection, length of the spinal needle, duration of the procedure, medications used for sedative purposes, local anesthesia, level of O_2 saturation in blood, appearance of the CFS, and adverse effects. These results confirm that LP is the best way to administer this medication in adolescent and young adults with later-onset SMA even in candidates with spinal bone deformities and respiratory failure mainly if the patient is managed under a multidisciplinary team.

Nusinersen is not available in Africa as yet but can be found in many European countries for all SMA types.

A few weeks ago, Sansone et al. [43] reported their experience and good results after studied 50 SMA patients treated with intrathecal nusinersen. They concluded that in spite of the severity of the disease and the age of patients, this treatment is feasible, safe, and suitable for SMA patients if they are managed by a good skilled team.

According to the information provided by Gidaro et al., a few weeks ago, in Australia, the commercial availability of the medication from the transition of expanded access programmed its right in corner. While in New Zealand, a broad access to this program is available, and in Canada, negotiators are discussing about the most convenient price at the present moment. However, some problems such as advanced age, patients with respiratory failure depending ventilator machine, and patients presenting spinal fusion still need to be solved [44].

As was mentioned before, the traditional LP for intrathecal administration of nusinersen can be impeded due to deformities of the spinal bone and orthopedic surgical procedures among other impediments commonly seen in SMA patients. However, the accumulated experiences from cervical myelograms serve to recommend this procedure as an ideal approach for cervical intrathecal administration of nusinersen, especially if it can be guided by ultrasound [45]. The same investigators studied 14 patients after the administration of nusinersen by cervical punctured guide by ultrasound with local anesthesia and found that all patients presented no major complications. One of the advantages of this technique is that general anesthesia is no required, and patients can be managed in real-time ultrasound guidance.

The most significant advantage to antisense oligonucleotide (ASO) therapeutics over other small molecule approaches is that acquisition of the target sequence provides immediate knowledge of putative complementary oligonucleotide therapeutics.

In 2019, Scoles et al. [46] described several therapeutic modalities with ASO and how they can be indicated for medical treatment of SMA, apart from the work done to develop novel ASO therapies looking for better results in the management of neurodegenerative disorders [46]. Novel advances of the genetic studies will allow distinguishing different genetic information for many neurological disorders. The mutated protein found and its chance to be placing into the cellular pathway will support a faster development of way for treatment. For the other hands, new opportunities for reliable treatment have been arising from the new capacities of targeting the disorder gene and RNAs. Among other procedures, to target the expression of RNA, some authors highlighted the utilization of ASOs to treat neurological problems. Treatment based on ASOs varies from 18 to 30 base pairs in length. These investigators changed expression of a target mRNA modifying splicing or by recruiting RNase H (cellular enzyme) that recognizes DNA: RNA hybrids causing target degradation [46].

Apart from nursinersen, other ASO therapeutics approved by FDA are eteplirsen to treat Duchene muscular dystrophy 2 and inotersen for managing patients presenting familial amyloid polyneuropathy. For treatment of Huntington disease, ASOs targeting HTT have been used [47]. As we and other authors reported in other publications, the treatment of choices for ALS is SOD1 and C9ORF72 [48, 49] and MAPT (TAU) in cases affected by Alzheimer disease [50]. Because most of the treatment with ASO does not cross the blood-brain barrier (BBB), it is necessary to administer it by injection into the intraventricular system in mouse and by intrathecal administration in humans.

Some investigators have mentioned that nucleic acids are prompt to nuclease degradation, and its protein binding is weak, leading to inefficient tissue uptake and unreliable use as drugs [26, 51].

Most of these changes modify the pharmacokinetic, pharmacodynamic, or endocytic uptake that controls the specific function of the proteins (cell surface) [51, 52].

Oligonucleotide chemistry, methoxyethyl oligonucleotide, constrained nucleic acids, Stereopure PS ASOs, Peptide nucleic acid, 5′-methylcytosine modification, target fate, mixed chemistry, and gapmers are aspects that are not discussed in this chapter and should be considered by interested readers on this matter. In order to get most complete information about it, we recommend checking the article of Scoles et al. [46].

ASOs are being used for some genetic etiology of ALS. Obviously, these biological pathways affecting the recognized mechanism of production of the disorder also modify the results when ASO is used [53].

2. Therapy with riluzole and edaravone

In 1994, the idea about the role of the excitatory amino acid neurotransmitter glutamate in the mechanism of production of ALS was prevalent. At that time, some investigators evaluated the safety and accuracy of the antiglutamate agent riluzole, at the dose of 100 mg daily, in patients presenting ALS. They studied 155 outpatients, and after 12 months of treatment, they found that 74% of the patients were still alive ($P = 0.014$), and the decrease of muscle power was remarkable in patients consuming riluzole compared with the control group (placebo). Therefore, they concluded that riluzole decreases the speed of progression in ALS patients, and it can prolong the survival period in patients presenting bulbar palsy [54].

Without doubt, nusinersen improves motor neuron function, but riluzole by acting on SK channels also causes similar results [55].

Since 1996, it is well known that one of the etiological pathogenesis of ALS is caused by neural damage due to glutamate excite-toxicity. Riluzole is a synthetic benzothiazole drug with glutamine antagonist activity [56, 57].

The first analyses, and at posteriori meta-analyses done on results obtained from controlled trials by randomization, confirm that riluzole extends survival by 2–3 months and augment the possibilities of an additional 12 months of survival by ~9%. Same authors reported improvements in media survival times over 76 weeks for an important number of ALS patients [58].

In 1995, oral riluzole was approved by FDA as part of the treatment of ALS. Riluzole is a well-known presynaptic glutamate release inhibitor, which can provide neural injury and prevent muscle-power worsening. Currently, this medication has been licensed to be prescribed in many places including the European Union [59].

The dose of 50 mg twice, to be taken 1 hour before meal or 2 hours after it, has been approved by the Institute for Health and Care Excellence since 2001 with good results [60].

One good news is that riluzole is now available in oral suspension (Teglutik®) which presentation (5 mg/ml) and has been shown its beneficial for patients presenting bulbar palsy with functional dysphagia allowing longer therapy [61, 62].

Not randomized controlled trials (RCTs) with riluzole for ALS patients have been performed.

However, other RCTs have been done for patients with cervical myelopathy, chronic psychosis, and autistic spectrum disorder [63–65].

Real-world evidence confirmed that an important prolongation of median survival times in ALS patients treated with riluzole is certain. Based on retrospective/prospective investigations done on large database, these authors concluded that patients under riluzole therapy had better prognosis than those without treatment, mainly at the first stage of the pathological process [58].

Brooks et al. studied two series of ALS patients: one group of 51 patients under riluzole treatment and another group of 241 patients without riluzole (before 1996) and a second series of 112 ALS patients' riluzole-treated and 65 nontreated patients (after 1996). These authors found that Cox analysis concluded that patients on treatment got an extension of survival ($P < 0.0001$) and even remarkable improvements in elderly people and patients in advanced stage. Therapy with riluzole provides a median extension of survival in affected patients between 40 and 72 weeks [66]. Survival benefit would be 36 weeks if patients are managed like prospective RCTs according to other researchers [67]. Based on Cox model technique, Mitchell et al. found that survival times are bigger in riluzole-treated ALS patients than nontreated cases (HR 0.20, $P < 0.001$) [68]. While other authors communicated that Cox multivariate analysis of therapy was related to a prolongation of survival at 48 weeks (HR 0.51, $P = 0.06$) [69].

Retrospective population-based studies on the effect of riluzole on survival of ALS patients done between 1999 and 2008 and made by Lee et al. concluded that Cox multivariate analysis ($n = 1149$) that riluzole provide a longer survival on treated-patients; unadjusted HR 0.32 ($P < 0.001$) and adjusted HR 0.34 ($P < 0.001$) [70].

Georgoulopoulou et al. and Knibb et al. conducted a prospective population-based study on the survival of 193 patients (between 2000 and 2009) and 575 cases (between 1990 and 2013) consuming riluzole, respectively. According to the Cox multivariate model used during the first series of participants riluzole-treated, they reached a prolonged survival and remarkable delay of pulmonary complications including patients with bulbar palsy and even those with affected four limbs, and the second series of cases riluzole-treated showed a slower progression to pulmonary involvement [71, 72].

Chen et al. also studied a group of ALS patients using the same methodology and concluded that the median survival time in cases riluzole-treated was 268 weeks compared to 256 weeks in nontreated cases (log-rank $P = 0.780$); HR 0.855 ($P = 0.167$) [73].

Based on meta-analysis of RCTs recently done and all data obtained up to date, riluzole prolonged survival in ALS cases by 8–12 weeks and augmented the chance of additional 52 weeks of survival by ~9%.

Other authors reported that riluzole-treated cases can increase their median survival by up to 76 weeks, after reviewing 10 clinical ALS databases with around ~6000 cases [58].

In a series of patients studied by Inoue-Shibui et al., riluzole therapy was interrupted in 20 cases among 92 patients [74]. The most common cause of discontinuation of riluzole was abnormal of liver enzymes (5.4%), followed by interstitial pneumonia, among other causes.

All adverse events happened within 24 weeks of the beginning of riluzole therapy, with 50% of the adverse events occurring within 2 weeks. In almost all patients, adverse events disappeared after stopping the treatment. In the real-world setting, riluzole has been well assimilated for long periods of up to 7 years or more [75].

Recently, two patients presenting recurrent pancreatitis were communicated to the medical literature. In both cases, the diagnosis was done within the first 3 months after initiated the treatment with riluzole [76], being another strong reason to highlight our recommendation about a careful observation of adverse events in the first 6 months of riluzole administration.

A few weeks ago, Jaiswal et al. also confirmed that riluzole delay progression of ALS in animal model based on their experiences and many experimental drug trials done over the past decades, but riluzole did not show similar results in human beings or results are still nonconcluded under Phase I–III trials, which are quite true, and riluzole is the only available medication with some benefits on survival [77]. Nevertheless, an antioxidant drug (edaravone) has been produced by Mitsubishi Tanabe Pharma, and its effectiveness in halting ALS progression during early stages has been found.

In 2015, edaravone (Ridicut) was launched for the management of patients with ischemic stroke at first and later for the treatment of ALS patients [78]. Edaravone is a drug with a free radical scavenger with no remarkable benefits in ALS patients according to Phase III clinical trial, but edaravone is also a strong antioxidant able to prevent oxidative stress leading to motor neuron fatal damage in ALS. These investigators found another study, which confirmed good therapeutic response to edaravone in diagnosed patients by revised diagnostic criteria (El Escorial) of MND/ALS. Other authors investigated the effect of intraperitoneal administration of edaravone in wobbler's mice and demonstrated that elevated dose (10 mg/kg) of edaravone therapy remarkable attenuated paresis and muscle contracture on the extremities and stopped denervation atrophy in the proximal muscles and degeneration in the cervical anterior horn cell neurons compared to control group. After large waiting period of 22 years, the Mitsubishi Tanabe Pharma America acquired an US FDA approval for edaravone (Radicava) in May 2017 for the therapeutic approach of ALS.

To low progression of MND/ALS, edaravone is a good indication according to the previous reports delivered to the medical literature. Recent phase three studies done on ALS patients treated with this medication did not confirm remarkable advantage in the Revised ALS Functional Rating score over the control group [79]. Between November 28, 2011 and September 3, 2014, the Writing Group [80] studied 213 cases and selected 192 candidates. Of these, 137 cases completed the first period for close observation: 69 were selected to be edaravone-treated (randomly), and 68 were assigned to control group to be treated with placebo also randomly, both series were included in the primary efficacy analysis. The results observed from the primary outcome demonstrated that the control group change −7.50 (0.66) in ALSFRS-R score compare with −5.01 (SE 0.64) in the group edaravone-treated. In favor of edaravone, the least-square mean confirmed a difference among two series of 2.49 (SE 0.76, 95% CI 0.99–33: P = 0.0013). These researchers concluded that edaravone works in a small subset of ALS patients who met criteria identified in post-hoc analysis of most recent Phase 3 studies, showing a remarkable diminish ALSFRS-R score compared with control group who received placebo. They also highlighted that there is no proof that edaravone might be efficient in a bigger series of ALS cases who do not meet the criteria [80]. The best way to administer edaravone (60 mg) is by slow IV infusion (2 hours duration) every 28 days. Edaravone has demonstrated its capacity to slow down the process of loss of motor function by 33% of ALS cases compared with control group. Being a powerful free radical scavenger, edaravone is able to inhibit nitration of tyrosine in the CSF and to improve the motor neuron cell activity in ALS mouse [81]. Unfortunately, there is no unanimous agreement about the positive effect of riluzole in patients presenting degenerative disorders. At the present moment, most of the neurology community agrees that riluzole is not a remarkable strong effect on the progression of ALS. Because the oxidative stress is considered to be involved in the pathology of ALS, almost all consider that the free radical scavenger edaravone may play a better relevant role for the treatment of cases presenting ALS. Without doubt, the first medication able to provide an efficient inhibition of motor neuron function deterioration in MND/ALS cases is edaravone if it is taken at early stage of this pathological disorder, but the lung function must be well assessed when a deterioration in the respiratory capacity is confirmed [82]. Most reports published in the medical literature show controversial benefits and safety about the edaravone treatment of ALS. Recently, Luo et al. [83] made a meta-analysis research to evaluate the accuracy and safety of edaravone as a therapy of choice for ALS, by searching PubMed, the Cochrane Library, and Embase from the inception of electronic data (April 2018), including randomized, double-blind, placebo-controlled trials reporting ALS cases receiving 60-mg IV edaravone or IV saline solution as placebo for 24 weeks. The study included 367 patients from three randomized controlled trials (183 patients on IV edaravone; 184 receiving IV saline solution). They arrived to the following conclusion: edaravone IV is a good treatment for ALS cases, with no remarkable side effects [83].

3. Other medications for MND

Although there is no available medicine to cure any clinical presentation of MND, during the first semester of this year (2019), a number of medications have been used to treat affected patients. Unfortunately, no remarkable results have been obtained, but some of them still show good action over this disease. In this chapter, we will deliver some comments about the results reached by some authors according to their report to the medical literature. The most common used medications are EH301, 5Fluoroucil, Tryptophan, RNS60, Rasagiline, Tirasemtiv, Aquaporin, Fasudil, and Lunasil.

de la Rubia et al. [84] evaluated the accuracy and feasibility of Elysium Health's candidate drug EH301 in ALS cases by a single-center, prospective, double-blind, randomized, placebo-controlled pilot study. Thirty-two ALS patients studied underwent for assessment during 4 months. Differences between EH301 and control group were evaluated based on their findings, and EH301 confirmed a remarkable slow progression of ALS compared with nontreated cases and even confirmed clinical benefits in many key outcome measures relative to their baseline.

Searching for drug candidates for ALS, Rando et al. investigated the action of anti-metabolite 5-fluorouracil (5-FU) administered by a single intraperitoneal injection at 150 mg/kg in SOD1G93A model of ALS. Un expectedly, the authors found that 5-FU (anti-cancer drug) increases survival delays of the disorder onset and improves motor function in ALS mice, but they were not able to demonstrate the mechanism of the beneficial 5-FU action in ALS mice. Despite of 5-FU did not improve the modulate motor neuron survival remarkably and did not improve reactive gliosis or change the muscle morphology, their findings recommended that a low dose of 5-FU or its analogs may have good effects on MND/ALS [85].

Other authors postulate that toxic gain of function, spread, and SOD1 misfolding is suggested as part of pathological mechanism of MND/ALS, but the nature of SOD1 toxicity has been hard to describe [86]. Only in SOD1 proteins from humans and other primates, and rarely in other species, a tryptophan residue at position 32 (W32) is predicted to be solvent exposed and to participate in SOD1 misfolding. DuVal et al. considered that W32 is influential in SOD1 acquiring toxicity, as it is known to be important in template-directed misfolding [86].

DuVal et al. highlighted the relevant influence of W32 on cases SOD1 toxicity to upper and lower motor neuron cells morphology and its activities. They assessed pharmaceutical targeting of the W32 residue for rescuing SOD1 toxicity [86]. When RNS60 is administered by IV infusion every 7 days and daily nebulization, it acts as a novel immune-modulator agent able to provide neuroprotective action in MND/ALS preclinical models. Paganoni et al. [87] studied 16 ALS patients during 23 weeks for safety and tolerability. Some investigations were done such as PBR28 positron emission tomography imaging and plasma biomarkers of inflammation. These authors did not find serious reactions, and no participants were removed from the study due to drug-related complications. At the present moment, a large, multicenter, Phase II trial of RNS60 is currently including cases to test the effects of RNS60 on MND/ALS biomarkers and disease deterioration based on the previous findings. They concluded that long-term RNS60 administered by IV infusion (as indicated) is well assimilated by patients and is also accurate [87]. In ALS, the prolong use of immune-modulating therapies has been showing not good results and did not help to understand how the immune system modifies disease outcome [88].

Rasagiline (monoamine oxidase B inhibitor) administered at 2 mg/day has a neuroprotective effect in MNS/ALS cases. In order to verify this postulate, Fernandez et al. performed a trial of 80 ALS patients from 10 hospitals in America. They did not identify any difference between Rasagiline-treated cases and the control group. Therefore, they assumed that Rasagiline did not change disease output compared with control group during 12 months of therapy. Rasagiline was well assimilated, and no serious adverse events were report.

Shefner et al. conducted a multinational clinical trial to study the accuracy of tirasemtiv (125 mg twice daily) using an escalating dosage protocol during 4 weeks [89]. Comparisons between two series of cases with ALS were performed. One group constituted by fast skeletal muscle troponin activator and a second control group by placebo. Of 744 candidates, 565 participants assimilated open-label tirasemtiv and were treated randomly. As a side effect of tirasemtiv, nausea, weight loss, dizziness, fatigue, and insomnia were more often seen. The frequency of severe side effects was seen equally on both series of cases. Obviously, tirasemtiv did not change the decline of slow vital capacity or remarkable impact secondary outcome assessment and weak tolerability of tirasemtiv may lead to poor effect on MND/ALS.

Aquaporin 4 (AQP4) is present in astrocytes in the nervous system as primary water channel and has been postulated to participate in a myriad of acute, chronic brain disorders and the incidence of MND/ALS. Depolarization of AQP4 causes degeneration of the upper and lower motor neurons via GLT-1, and suppressions increase recovery of motor activity in MND/ALS cases probable due to NGF. No clinical trial targeting AQP4 has been done up to date [90].

Studies made with Fasudil (30 mg for IV application) have shown good results in cell culture and animal research of MND/ALS. This medication is a Rho kinase (ROCK) inhibitor, which has been used in Japan (1995) for the management of Reynaud's syndrome, pulmonary hypertension, and vasospasm secondary to subarachnoid hemorrhage, angina pectoris, and also to treat complications from high blood pressure. Currently, some authors are looking for efficacy, safety and tolerability of a ROCK-ALS of fasudil in MND/ALS cases that started patient recruitment in 2019 [91]. ROCK (serine/threonine kinase) is a novel medication to target for neurodegenerative brain disorders, and it has two isoforms: ROCK1 is mainly for the peripheral nervous system, and ROCK2 is expressed preferentially in nervous central system [92]. Levels of ROCK augment according to age and tissue of MND/ALS cases. Some authors also confirmed increased levels of ROCK2 and downstream targets LIMK1 and coiling [93]. Fasudil also modifies microglia activity [91]. Main side effect of fasudil is intraparenchymal hemorrhage. Nevertheless, in studied population of cases with subarachnoid hemorrhage, the incidence of bleeding did not differ remarkably from the control group. Therefore, hemorrhage is not an expected complication, and it will not put in risk the life in selected patient. Cases with past medical history of intraparenchymal bleeding, congenital or acquire aneurysms or Moyamoya disease should not be included in the therapeutic group.

Lingor et al. confirmed that ROCK-MND/ALS clinical trial provides a well-tolerated, safe, and accurate way of treatment. The biomarker collection associated with this study will deliver additional data as indicators of progression. Finally, we comment about Lunasin a soy peptide that modify histone acetylation in vitro joined to single MND/ALS effect but no remarkable activity on histone acetylation or disorder deterioration in 50 participants treated during 5.5 months by Bedlack et al. [94]. Excellent retention and adherence have been found but not better results than riluzole or edaravone.

As a result of the great interest showed by investigators and participants on different studies done during the first half of this year (2019), today we can see an important number of other therapeutic procedures also looking for the best management of ALS patients. This modality ranges from physical exercises to acupuncture including other choices such as stem cell therapy, treatment for sialorrhea, and spasticity, among others.

In our times, many healthy people do physical exercises on regular basis; some do exercise for slimming purposes, others for prophylactic treatment, rehabilitation, and so forth.

Unfortunately, due to lack of space, these topics will not be included in this chapter.

After reviewing the most recent studies published in the medical literature, we concluded that we still have no curative treatment for MND patients, but a promising future is forthcoming.

Author details

Humberto Foyaca Sibat* and Lourdes de Fátima Ibañez Valdés
Department of Neurology, Faculty of Health Sciences, Nelson Mandela Academic Central Hospital, Walter Sisulu University, Mthatha, South Africa

*Address all correspondence to: humbertofoyacasibat@gmail.com

References

[1] Foyaca Sibat H, de Fátima Ibañez Valdés L. Chapter I. Introduction to update in amyotrophic lateral sclerosis and review of this condition in sportsmen. Update in Amyotrophic Lateral Sclerosis. In: Sibat HF, editor. Rijeka: IntechOpen; 2016. Available from: http://www.intechopen.com/myprofile/index/dashboard http://dx.doi.org/10.5772/64608

[2] Dupuis L, Petersen Å, Weydt P. Thermoregulation in amyotrophic lateral sclerosis. Handbook of Clinical Neurology. 2018;**157**:749-760. DOI: 10.1016/B978-0-444-64074-1.00046-X

[3] Mehta P, Kaye W, Raymond J, Punjani R, Larson T, Cohen J, et al. Prevalence of amyotrophic lateral sclerosis—United States, 2015. Morbidity and Mortality Weekly Report. 2018;**67**(46):1285-1289. DOI: 10.15585/mmwr.mm6746a1

[4] Lopez-Vega JM, Calleja J, Combarros O, Polo JM, Berciano J. Motor neuron disease in Cantabria. Acta Neurologica Scandinavica. 1988;**77**:1-5

[5] Zarranz JJ. Neurología. 4th ed. Madrid: Elsevier; 2008

[6] Amato A, Russell J. Neuromuscular Disorders. McGrawHill: China; 2008

[7] Dunckley T, Huentelman MJ, Craig DW, Pearson JV, Szelinger S, Joshipura K, et al. Whole-genome analysis of sporadic amyo-trophic lateral sclerosis. The New England Journal of Medicine. 2007;**357**:775-788

[8] Van Es MA, van Vught PW, Blauw HM, Franke L, Saris CG, van Den BL, et al. Genetic variation in DPP6 is associatedwith susceptibility to amyotrophic lateral sclerosis. Nature Genetics. 2008;**40**:29-31

[9] Van Es MA, van Vught PW, Blauw HM, Franke L, Saris CG, Andersen PM, et al. ITPR2 as a susceptibility gene insporadic amyotrophic lateral sclerosis: A genome-wide asso-ciation study. Lancet Neurology. 2007;**6**:869-877

[10] DeJesus-Hernandez M, Mackenzie IR, Boeve BF, Boxer AL, Baker M, Rutherford NJ, et al. Expanded GGGGCC hexa-nucleotide repeat in noncoding region of C9ORF72 causeschromosome 9p-linked FTD and ALS. Neuron. 2011;**72**:245-256

[11] Renton AE, Majounie E, Waite A, Simon-Sanchez J, Rollinson S, Gibbs JR, et al. A hexanucleotide repeat expansion in C9ORF72is the cause of chromosome 9p21-linked ALS-FTD. Neuron. 2011;**72**:257-268

[12] Thompson AG, Gray E, Thézénas ML, Charles PD, Evetts S, Hu MT, et al. Cerebrospinal fluid macrophage biomarkers in amyotrophic lateral sclerosis. Journal Annals of Neurology. 2018;**83**(2):258-268. DOI: 10.1002/ana.25143. [Epub: 9 February 2018]

[13] Sancho J, Servera E, Bañuls P, Marín J. Effectiveness of assisted and unassisted cough capacity in amyotrophic lateral sclerosis patients. Amyotrophic Lateral Sclerosis and Frontotemporal Degeneration. 2017;**18**(7-8):498-504. DOI: 10.1080/21678421.2017.1335324. [Epub: 9 June 2017]

[14] Allodi I, Nijssen J, Benitez JA, Schweingruber C, Fuchs A, Bonvicini G, et al. Modeling motor neuron resilience in ALS using stem cells. Stem Cell Reports. 2019;**6711**(19)30131-30136. DOI: 10.1016/j.stemcr.2019.04.009

[15] Edmond EC, Stagg CJ, Turner MR. Therapeutic non-invasive brain stimulation in amyotrophic lateral sclerosis: rationale, methods and

experience. The Journal of Neurology, Neurosurgery, and Psychiatry. 2019. pii: jnnp-2018-320213. DOI: 10.1136/jnnp-2018-320213

[16] de Alcântara C, Cruzeiro MM, França MC Jr, Camargos ST, de Souza LC. Amyotrophic lateral sclerosis type 8 is not a pure motor disease: Evidence from a neuropsychological and behavioural study. Journal of Neurology. 2019. DOI: 10.1007/s00415-019-09369-y

[17] Ando S, Funato M, Ohuchi K, Inagaki S, Sato A, Seki J, et al. The protective effects of Levetiracetam on a human iPSCs-derived spinal muscular atrophy model. Neurochemical Research. 2019. DOI: 10.1007/s11064-019-02814-4

[18] Bozorg Qomi S, Asghari A, Salmaninejad A, Mojarrad M. Spinal muscular atrophy and common therapeutic advances. Fetal and Pediatric Pathology. 2019;**38**:1-13. DOI: 10.1080/15513815.2018. 1520374

[19] Peikert K, Naumann M, Günther R, Wegner F, Hermann A. Off-label treatment of 4 amyotrophic lateral sclerosis patients with 4-Aminopyridine. Journal of Clinical Pharmacology. 2019. DOI: 10.1002/jcph.1437

[20] Neil EE, Bisaccia EK. Nusinersen: A novel antisense oligonucleotide for the treatment of spinal muscular atrophy. Journal of Pediatric Pharmacology and Therapeutics. 2019;**24**(3):194-203. DOI: 10.5863/1551-6776-24.3.194

[21] Sugarman EA, Nagan N, Zhu H, et al. Pan-ethnic carrier screening and prenatal diagnosis for spinal muscular atrophy: Clinical laboratory analysis of >72,400 specimens. European Journal of Human Genetics. 2012;**20**:27-32

[22] Lunn MR, Wang CH. Spinal muscular atrophy. Lancet. 2008;**371**:2120-2133

[23] Saffari A, Kölker S, Hoffmann GF, Weiler M, Ziegler A. Novel challenges in spinal muscular atrophy—How to screen and whom to treat? Annals of Clinical Translational Neurology. 2019;**6**(1):197-205

[24] Finkel RS, Mercuri E, Darras BT, et al. Nusinersen versus sham control in infantile-onset spinal muscular atrophy. The New England Journal of Medicine. 2017;**377**:1723-1732. [PubMed] [Google Scholar]

[25] Mercuri E, Darras BT, Chiriboga CA, et al. Nusinersen versus sham control in later-onset spinal muscular atrophy. The New England Journal of Medicine. 2018;**378**:625-635

[26] Bennett CF, Swayze EE. RNA targeting therapeutics: Molecular mechanisms of antisense oligonucleotides as a therapeutic platform. Annual Review of Pharmacology and Toxicology. 2010;**50**:259-293

[27] Campbell MA, Wengel J. Locked vs. unlocked nucleic acids (LNA vs. UNA): Contrasting structures work towards common therapeutic goals. Chemical Society Reviews. 2011;**40**:5680-5689

[28] Elmén J, Thonberg H, Ljungberg K, et al. Locked nucleic acid (LNA) mediated improvements in siRNA stability and functionality. Nucleic Acids Research. 2005;**33**:439-447

[29] Mouawia H, Saker A, Jais JP, et al. Circulating trophoblastic cells provide genetic diagnosis in 63 fetuses at risk for cystic fibrosis or spinal muscular atrophy. Reproductive Biomedicine Online. 2012;**25**:508-520

[30] Parks M, Court S, Bowns B, et al. Non-invasive prenatal diagnosis of spinal muscular atrophy by relative haplotype dosage. European Journal of Human Genetics. 2017;**25**:416-422

[31] Bianchi DW, Chiu RWK. Sequencing of circulating cell-free DNA during pregnancy. The New England Journal of Medicine. 2018;**379**:464-473

[32] Iwamoto N, Butler DCD, Svrzikapa N, et al. Control of phosphorothioate stereochemistry substantially increases the efficacy of antisense oligonucleotides. Nature Biotechnology. 2017;**35**:845-851

[33] Wan WB, Migawa MT, Vasquez G, et al. Synthesis, biophysical properties and biological activity of second-generation antisense oligonucleotides containing chiral phosphorothioate linkages. Nucleic Acids Research. 2014;**42**:13456-13468

[34] Kaihatsu K, Janowski BA, Corey DR. Recognition of chromosomal DNA by PNAs. Chemistry & Biology. 2004;**11**:749-758

[35] Stein CA. The experimental use of antisense oligonucleotides: A guide for the perplexed. The Journal of Clinical Investigation. 2001;**108**:641-644

[36] Krieg AM, Yi AK, Matson S, et al. CpG motifs in bacterial DNA trigger direct B-cell activation. Nature. 1995;**374**:546-549

[37] Drygin D, Barone S, Bennett CF. Sequence-dependent cytotoxicity of second-generation oligonucleotides. Nucleic Acids Research. 2004;**32**:6585-6594

[38] Aartsma-Rus A. FDA approval of nusinersen for spinal muscular atrophy makes 2016 the year of splice modulating oligonucleotides. Nucleic Acid Therapeutics. 2017;**27**:67-69

[39] Chiriboga CA, Swoboda KJ, Darras BT, et al. Results from a phase 1 study of nusinersen (ISIS-SMN(Rx)) in children with spinal muscular atrophy. Neurology. 2016;**86**:890-897

[40] Luu KT, Norris DA, Gunawan R, et al. Population pharmacokinetics of nusinersen in the cerebral spinal fluid and plasma of pediatric patients with spinal muscular atrophy following intrathecal administrations. Journal of Clinical Pharmacology. 2017;**57**:1031-1041

[41] Finkel RS, Chiriboga CA, Vajsar J, et al. Treatment of infantile-onset spinal muscular atrophy with nusinersen: A phase 2, open-label, dose-escalation study. Lancet. 2016;**388**:3017-3026

[42] Wurster CD, Winter B, Wollinsky K, Ludolph AC, Uzelac Z, Witzel S, et al. Intrathecal administration of nusinersen in adolescent and adult SMA type 2 and 3 patients. Journal of Neurology. 2019;**266**(1):183-194. DOI: 10.1007/s00415-018-9124-0

[43] Sansone VA, Albamonte E, Salmin F, Casiraghi J, Pirola A, Bettinelli M, et al. Intrathecal nusinersen treatment for SMA in a dedicated neuromuscular clinic: An example of multidisciplinary and integrated care. Neurological Sciences. 2019;**40**(2):327-332. DOI: 10.1007/s10072-018-3622-9

[44] Gidaro T, Servais L. Nusinersen treatment of spinal muscular atrophy: Current knowledge and existing gaps. Developmental Medicine and Child Neurology. 2019;**61**(1):19-24. DOI: 10.1111/dmcn.14027

[45] Ortiz CB, Kukreja KU, Lotze TE, Chau A. Ultrasound-guided cervical puncture for nusinersen administration in adolescents. Pediatric Radiology. 2019;**49**(1):136-140. DOI: 10.1007/s00247-018-4240-7

[46] Scoles DR, Minikel EV, Pulst SM. Antisense oligonucleotides. Neurology: Genetics. 2019;**5**(2):e323. DOI: 10.1212/NXG.0000000000000323

[47] van Roon-Mom WMC, Roos RAC, de Bot ST. Dose-dependent lowering

of mutant huntingtin using antisense oligonucleotides in Huntington disease patients. Nucleic Acid Therapeutics. 2018;**28**:59-62

[48] McCampbell A, Cole T, Wegener AJ, et al. Antisense oligonucleotides extend survival and reverse decrement in muscle response in ALS models. The Journal of Clinical Investigation. 2018;**128**:3558-3567

[49] Ly CV, Miller TM. Emerging antisense oligonucleotide and viral therapies for amyotrophic lateral sclerosis. Current Opinion in Neurology. 2018;**31**:648-654

[50] DeVos SL, Goncharoff DK, Chen G, et al. Antisense reduction of tau in adult mice protects against seizures. The Journal of Neuroscience. 2013;**33**:12887-12897

[51] Crooke ST, Wang S, Vickers TA, Shen W, Liang XH. Cellular uptake and trafficking of antisense oligonucleotides. Nature Biotechnology. 2017;**35**:230-237

[52] Geary RS, Norris D, Yu R, Bennett CF. Pharmacokinetics, biodistribution and cell uptake of antisense oligonucleotides. Advanced Drug Delivery Reviews. 2015;**87**:46-51

[53] Klim JR, Vance C, Scotter EL. Antisense oligonucleotide therapies for amyotrophic lateral sclerosis: Existing and emerging targets. The International Journal of Biochemistry & Cell Biology. 2019;**110**:149-153. DOI: 10.1016/ j.biocel. 2019.03.009

[54] Bensimon G, Lacomblez L, Meininger V. A controlled trial of riluzole in amyotrophic lateral sclerosis. ALS/Riluzole study group. The New England Journal of Medicine. 1994;**330**(9):585-591

[55] Dimitriadi M, Kye MJ, Kalloo G, Yersak JM, Sahin M, Hart AC. The neuroprotective drug riluzole acts via small conductance Ca^{2+}-activated K^+ channels to ameliorate defects in spinal muscular atrophy models. The Journal of Neuroscience. 2013;**33**(15):6557-6562. DOI: 10.1523/JNEUROSCI.1536-12.2013

[56] Brayfield A, editor. Martindale: The Complete Drug Reference. 37th ed. London, England, UK: Pharmaceutical Press; 2011. Available from https:// www.medicinescomplete.com [Accessed: 14 May 2019]

[57] NCBI (National Center for Biotechnology Information). PubChem Compound Database; CID = 5070 (Riluzole) [webpage on the Internet]. Available from: https://pubchem. ncbi.nlm.nih.gov/compound/ riluzole#section=Top [Accessed: 15 May 2019]

[58] Hinchcliffe M, Smith A. Riluzole: Real-world evidence supports significant extension of median survival times in patients with amyotrophic lateral sclerosis. Degenerative Neurological and Neuromuscular Disease. 2017;7:61-70. DOI: 10.2147/ DNND.S135748

[59] Gaber TA-ZK, Mehmood Z, Siringwani H. Riluzole. Progress in Neurology and Psychiatry. 2016;**20**:32-33

[60] NICE (National Institute for Clincal Excellence) (Technology Appraisal Guidance) TA20. Guidance on the Use of Riluzole (Rilutek) for the Treatment of Motor Neurone Disease. 2001. Available from: https://www.nice.org.uk/ Guidance/ta20 [Accessed: 19 May 2019]

[61] Dyer AM, Smith A. Riluzole 5 mg/ mL oral suspension: For optimized drug delivery in amyotrophic lateral sclerosis. Drug Design, Development and Therapy. 2017;**11**:59-64

[62] Keating GM. Riluzole oral suspension in amyotrophic lateral

sclerosis: A guide to its use. Drugs & Therapy Perspectives. 2016;**32**(7):282-286

[63] Ghaleiha A, Mohammadi E, Mohammadi M-R, et al. Riluzole as an adjunctive therapy to risperidone for the treatment of irritability in children with autistic disorder: A double-blind, placebo-controlled, randomized trial. Pediatric Drugs. 2013;**15**(6):505-514

[64] Rajasekaran S, Aiyer SN, Shetty AP, Kanna RM, Maheswaran A, Shetty JY. Effectiveness of riluzole as a pharmacotherapeutic treatment option for early cervical myelopathy: A double-blinded, placebo-controlled randomised controlled trial. European Spine Journal. 2016;**25**(6):1830-1835

[65] Farokhnia M, Sabzabadi M, Pourmahmoud H, et al. A double-blind, placebo controlled, randomized trial of riluzole as an adjunct to risperidone for treatment of negative symptoms in patients with chronic schizophrenia. Psychopharmacology. 2014;**231**(3):533-542

[66] Brooks BR, Belden DS, Roelke K, et al. Survival in non-riluzole treated amyotrophic lateral sclerosis (ALS)—Motor neuron disease (MND) patients with disease onset before and since 1996 is identical: A clinic-based epidemiological study. Amyotrophic Lateral Sclerosis and Other Motor Neuron Disorders. 2001;**2**:60-61

[67] Turner MR, Bakker M, Sham P, Shaw CE, Leigh PN, Al-Chalabi A. Prognostic modelling of therapeutic interventions in amyotrophic lateral sclerosis. Amyotrophic Lateral Sclerosis and Other Motor Neuron Disorders. 2002;**3**(1):15-21

[68] Mitchell JD, O'Brien MR, Joshi M. Audit of outcomes in motor neuron disease (MND) patients treated with riluzole. Amyotrophic Lateral Sclerosis. 2006;7(2):67-71

[69] Zoccolella S, Beghi E, Palagano G, et al. SLAP registry Riluzole and amyotrophic lateral sclerosis survival: A population-based study in southern Italy. European Journal of Neurology. 2007;**14**(3):262-268

[70] Lee CT-C, Chiu Y-W, Wang K-C, et al. Riluzole and prognostic factors in amyotrophic lateral sclerosis long-term and short-term survival: A population-based study of 1149 cases in Taiwan. Journal of Epidemiology. 2013;**23**(1):35-40

[71] Georgoulopoulou E, Fini N, Vinceti M, et al. The impact of clinical factors, riluzole and therapeutic interventions on ALS survival: A population-based study in Modena, Italy. Amyotrophic Lateral Sclerosis and Frontotemporal Degeneration. 2013;**14**(5-6):338-345 [PubMed] [Google Scholar]

[72] Knibb JA, Keren N, Kulka A, et al. A clinical tool for predicting survival in ALS. Journal of Neurology, Neurosurgery, and Psychiatry. 2016;**87**(12):1361-1367

[73] Chen L, Liu X, Tang L, Zhang N, Fan D. Long-term use of riluzole could improve the prognosis of sporadic amyotrophic lateral sclerosis patients: A real-world cohort study in China. Frontiers in Aging Neuroscience. 2016;**8**:246

[74] Inoue-Shibui A, Kato M, Suzuki N, Kobayashi J, Takai Y, Izumi R, et al. Interstitial pneumonia and other adverse events in riluzole-administered amyotrophic lateral sclerosis patients: A retrospective observational study. BMC Neurology. 2019;**19**:72

[75] Fang T, Al Khleifat A, Meurgey JH, Jones A, Leigh PN, Bensimon G, et al. Stage at which riluzole treatment prolongs survival in patients with amyotrophic lateral sclerosis: A retrospective analysis of data from

a dose-ranging study. The Lancet Neurology. 2018;**17**(5):416-422

[76] Falcão de Campos C, de Carvalho M. Riluzole-induced recurrent pancreatitis. Journal of Clinical Neuroscience. 2017;**45**:153-154

[77] Jaiswal MK. Riluzole and edaravone: A tale of two amyotrophic lateral sclerosis drugs. Medicinal Research Reviews. 2019;**39**(2):733-748. DOI: 10.1002/med.21528

[78] Ikeda K, Iwasaki Y. Edaravone, a free radical scavenger, delayed symptomatic and pathological progression of motor neuron disease in the wobbler mouse. PLoS One. 2015;**10**(10):e0140316. DOI: 10.1371/journal.pone.0140316

[79] Lipman R, Kuskel R. Edaravone a novel neuroprotective agent. Journal of Neurology, Neurosurgery, and Psychiatry. 2017;**89**:144-151

[80] Writing Group; Edaravone (MCI-186) ALS 19 Study Group. Safety and efficacy of edaravone in well defined patients with amyotrophic lateral sclerosis: A randomized, double-blind, placebo-controlled trial. Lancet Neurology. 2017;**16**(7):505-512. DOI: 10.1016/S1474-4422(17)30115-1

[81] Bhandari R, Kuhad A, Kuhad A. Edaravone: A new hope for deadly amyotrophic lateral sclerosis. Drugs of Today (Barcelona, Spain: 1998). 2018;**54**(6):349-360. DOI: 10.1358/dot.2018.54.6.2828189

[82] Yoshino H. Edaravone for the treatment of amyotrophic lateral sclerosis. Expert Review of Neurotherapeutics. 2019;**19**(3):185-193. DOI: 10.1080/14737175.2019.1581610

[83] Luo L, Song Z, Li X, Huiwang, Zeng Y, Qinwang, et al. Efficacy and safety of edaravone in treatment of amyotrophic lateral sclerosis-a systematic review and meta-analysis. Neurological Sciences. 2019;**40**(2):235-241. DOI: 10.1007/s10072-018-3653-2

[84] de la Rubia JE, Drehmer E, Platero JL, Benlloch M, Caplliure-Llopis J, Villaron-Casales C, et al. Efficacy and tolerability of EH301 for amyotrophic lateral sclerosis: a randomized, double-blind, placebo-controlled human pilot study. Amyotrophic Lateral Sclerosis and Frontotemporal Degeneration. 2019;**20**(1-2):115-122. DOI: 10.1080/21678421.2018.1536152

[85] Rando A, de la Torre M, Martinez-Muriana A, Zaragoza P, Musaro A, Hernández S, et al. Chemotherapeutic agent 5-fluorouracil increases survival of SOD1 mouse model of ALS. PLoS One. 2019;**14**(1):e0210752

[86] DuVal MG, Hinge VK, Snyder N, Kanyo R, Bratvold J, Pokrishevsky E, et al. Tryptophan 32 mediates SOD1 toxicity in a in vivo motor neuron model of ALS and is a promising target for small molecule therapeutics. Neurobiology of Disease. 2019;**124**:297-310. DOI: 10.1016/j.nbd.2018.11.025

[87] Paganoni S, Alshikho MJ, Luppino S, Chan J, Pothier L, Schoenfeld D, et al. A pilot trial of RNS60 in amyotrophic lateral sclerosis. Muscle & Nerve. 2019;**59**(3):303-308. DOI: 10.1002/mus.26385

[88] Wosiski-Kuhn M, Lyon MS, Caress J, Milligan C. Inflammation, immunity, and amyotrophic lateral sclerosis: II. Immune-modulating therapies. Muscle & Nerve. 2019;**59**(1):23-33. DOI: 10.1002/mus.26288

[89] Shefner JM, Cudkowicz ME, Hardiman O, Cockroft BM, Lee JH, Malik FI, et al. A phase III trial of tirasemtiv as a potential treatment for amyotrophic lateral sclerosis. Amyotrophic Lateral Sclerosis and Frontotemporal Degeneration. 2019;**27**:1-9. DOI: 10.1080/21678421.2019.1612922

[90] Zou S, Lan YL, Wang H, Zhang B, Sun YG. The potential roles of aquaporin 4 in amyotrophic lateral sclerosis. Neurological Sciences. 2019. DOI: 10.1007/s10072-019-03877-5

[91] Lingor P, Weber M, Camu W, Friede T, Hilgers R, Leha A, et al. Tolerability and efficacy of the Rho kinase (ROCK) inhibitor fasudil in amyotrophic lateral sclerosis. Frontiers in Neurology. 2019;**10**:293

[92] Koch J-C, Tatenhorst L, Roser AE, Saal KA, Tönges L, Lingor P. ROCK inhibition in models of neurodegeneration and its potential for clinical translation. Pharmacology & Therapeutics. 2018;**189**(C):1-21. DOI: 10.1016/j.pharmthera.2018.03.008

[93] Conti A, Riva N, Pesca M, Iannaccone S, Cannistraci CV, Corbo M, et al. Increased expression of myosin binding protein H in the skeletal muscle of amyotrophic lateral sclerosis patients. Biochimica et Biophysica Acta. 2014;**1842**:99-106. DOI: 10.1016/j.bbadis.2013.10.013

[94] Bedlack RS, Wicks P, Vaughan T, Opie A, Blum R, Dios A, et al. Lunasin does not slow ALS progression: Results of an open-label, single-center, hybrid-virtual 12-month trial. Amyotrophic Lateral Sclerosis and Frontotemporal Degeneration. 2019;**21**:1-9. DOI: 10.1080/21678421.2018.1556698

Section 2

Novel Information on Amyoyrophic Lateral Sclerosis and Spinal Muscular Atrophic

Chapter 5

Novel Aspects on Motor Neuron Disease: The Recent Genetic Studies on ALS

Junling Wang

Abstract

At present, with the advanced affordable genetic testing, the rate of discovering amyotrophic lateral sclerosis (ALS)-related genes rapidly increases. These genetic findings provide new insights into therapies that target genetic subset of ALS. However, the research on the genetic and environmental causes of ALS is still in the early stage. In this chapter, we review the current understanding of ALS-related genes and summarize the worldwide ALS distribution feature by the frequency of occurrence in different regions. We summarize the advances in genetic testing and counseling for ALS. Based on the increase in genetic testing, we believe that the ALS patients and families would be benefited from our studies in the near future.

Keywords: ALS, genetic frequency features, GWAS, genetic testing, genetic counseling, genetic therapy

1. Introduction

Amyotrophic lateral sclerosis (ALS) is an adult onset and generally fatal neurodegenerative disease characterized by progressive weakness and atrophy of voluntary skeletal muscles due to dysfunction and death of upper and lower motor neurons. Onset typically occurs between 60 and 69 years of age, with wide-range severity. About 90% of cases are sporadic amyotrophic lateral sclerosis (SALS), while familial amyotrophic lateral sclerosis (FALS) accounts for the remaining 10% cases [1]. The pathogenesis of ALS remains obscure, but genetic mutations have been accounted for several impaired cellular and molecular mechanisms and, thus, provide clues for potential therapeutic strategies.

The superoxide dismutase 1 (*SOD1*), identified in 1993, was the first gene discovered to be associated with ALS. Subsequently, several gene mutations that have been identified to cause ALS. Till 2018, more than 180 genes have been identified as causative genes or related genes of ALS. Many of these genes are related to metabolism, trafficking of RNA, and chromatin, including *C9orf 72*, *TDP43*, *FUS*, *TAF15*, *ELP3*, *ANG*, *hnRNPA1*, and *hnRNPA2B1* [2]. Some genes are involved in conformational instability and aggregation of proteins, such as *SOD1*, *VCP*, *OPTN*, and *UBQLN2*; others are related to axonal and cytoskeletal biology, such as *PFN1*, *DCTN1*, *TUBA4A*, and *EPHA4* [2].

In most cases, FALS is inherited in the dominant pattern and the penetrance is associated with age. It has been observed that the differences of age onset and disease progression within and between ALS families are significant. In addition, some ALS is recessive inherited, such as *OPTN*, *SPG11*, *FUS*, and *SOD1* (definite, Asp90Ala homozygous mutation), and *UBQLN2 associated ALS* is X-linked dominant inherited. Besides causative genes, multiple genetic variants interact simultaneously to increase ALS susceptibility. Considering oligogenic manner of ALS described by some researchers, many ALS patients may not appear to be familial in a conventional Mendelian manner. Therefore, the oligogenic manner may underlie the apparently sporadic form of the disease [3].

Some ALS caused by specific genetic mutations exhibit unique clinical characteristics. For example, ALS associated with *SPG11* and *ALS3* has clinical features of early onset and slow progression. *SPG11* mutations were identified in autosomal recessive juvenile ALS [4], and the patients with *ALS3* mutations have an early onset of approximately 45 years and the average disease duration about 5 years.

Recently, progress in gene discovery and technology has both complicated and empowered the process of genetic testing options, which may help neurological clinicians and ALS patients to understand the pathogenesis of ALS, and then provide genetic counseling for family members, allow accurate risk assessment, and open the door for genotype-specific treatments. As the genetic basis of the remainder of FALS, and potentially SALS, is unraveled, genetic testing and counseling will become increasingly vital and should be incorporated into the routine management of ALS [4–6].

2. Recent advances in ALS gene map

2.1 *SOD1*

The superoxide dismutase 1 (*SOD1*), located in 21q22, was discovered in 1993. Up to date, more than 180 mutations have been described to be associated with ALS, while most of these mutations are missense mutations. Its mutation probability accounts for 20% of FALS cases and 1–2% of SALS cases [1, 2, 7, 8].

2.2 *C9orf 72*

The *C9orf 72*, located in 9p21.2, was discovered in 2011. The protein encoded by *C9orf 72* is mainly related to autophagy, endosomal transport, and immune function. According to statistics, about 40–50% of FALS and 10% of SALS carried the *C9orf 72* expanded alleles. The pathogenic alleles of *C9orf 72* may have hundreds or even thousands of the GGGGCC hexanucleotide repeats. A large number of clinical investigations have shown that about 700–1600 GGGGCC hexanucleotide repeats are inserted into the intron located between the two untranslated optional exons 1a and 1b of the *C9orf 72* gene [1–3, 9, 10].

2.3 *FUS*

The FUS RNA-binding protein (*FUS*) gene, discovered in 2009, was mapped in 16p11.2.

Mutations in *FUS* are observed in 4% of FALS and 1% of SALS. At present, more than 79 mutations have been described, predominantly in the 3′ region encoding an arginine/glycine-rich region and a NLS domain (nuclear localization signal). FUS protein, essentially localized in the nucleus, regulates RNA processing, splicing, and mRNA trafficking. Mutant FUS localized to cytoplasmic stress granules (SGs) and interacted with the stress granule protein PABP in an RNA-dependent manner resulting in mislocalization of the wildtype protein to stress granules [7–9, 11].

2.4 *CCNF*

CCNF, located in 16p13.3, encoding the cyclin F, was first reported in 2016. The mutation of *CCNF* accounts for approximately 4% of FALS and 2% of SALS [7].

CCNF protein is a kind of kithe cell cyclin, involved in the regular of cell cycle transitions by activating cyclin-dependent protein kinases. Furthermore, it is the substrate recognition component of the Skp1-cullin-F-box E3 ubiquitin ligase complex. The neurons of the over-expressed mutant CCNF showed an increase in protein-labeled proteins, including TDP43. It indicates that mutated-CCNF protein interfere the proteasome degradation pathway by using traversing protein abnormalities to mark all proteins or inhibiting transferring transprotein-labeled proteins to proteasome complexes. This finding suggests that the *CCNF* mutation may cause abnormal protein homeostasis, which may be exacerbated by TDP43 protein disease.

Therefore, enhancing protein removal or reducing ubiquitin may be a feasible treatment [1, 3].

2.5 *TIA1*

The *TIA1* gene, located in 2p13.3, encodes an RNA-binding protein involved in splicing regulation and translational repression. The mutations in *TIA1* were identified in 2.2% of FALS and 0.4% of SALS [7]. TIA1 protein is a key component of SGs, cytoplasmic foci sequester untranslated mRNAs upon different types of cellular stress, and the low complexity domain (LCD) region of TIA1 plays a central role in promoting SGs assembly. A heterozygous founder mutation (E384K) in the LCD was first reported in Swedish/Finnish patients as the cause of Welander distal myopathy (WDM). Recently, a mutation (p.P362L) in *TIA1* affecting a highly conserved residue in the LCD was identified as one cause of ALS/ALS-FTD [12].

2.6 *TBK1*

The TANK-binding kinase 1 (*TBK1*) gene, located in 12q14.2, was discovered in 2015 [7]. The protein encoded by this gene is similar to the IκB kinase and can mediate NFκb activation in response to certain growth factors. The *TBK1* mutations were found in approximately 1% of FALS and 1% of SALS. The clinical phenotypes associated with the *TBK1* mutation are heterogeneous, with different ages at onset, different progressions, and irregular survival times.

Some patients also reported with extrapyramidal, ataxia, or psychosis. Neuropathological examination of central nervous system (CNS) tissues from patients with *TBK1* mutations revealed that SQSTM1/p62- and TDP-43-positive inclusion bodies which can indicate abnormalities in TDP-43 protein aggregation and protein clearance pathways [1, 2, 4, 5].

2.7 *TARDBP*

The *TARDBP* (trans-activation element DNA-binding protein), located in 1p36.22, was discovered in 2008 [5].

The *TARDBP* gene mutation was found in 5% of FALS cases and 1% in SALS cases. Till now, more than 50 different mutations have been identified [9]. Except for D169G, a majority of these mutations are located in the 3′ region encoding a glycine-rich domain in its product, TDP-43. ALS patients carrying *TARDBP* gene mutations normally exhibit a classical ALS phenotype and rare dementia, they also have earlier disease onset, with upper limb onset being more common and compatible with a longer life. Most of TDP-43 is expressed in nucleus, involved in RNA metabolism in many ways—transcriptional regulation, splicing, mRNA stabilization (including its own transcripts), and microRNA processing. TDP43 also regulates axonal transport and neuronal plasticity. In ALS, TDP-43 is often observed in cytoplasm. The pathogenesis of TDP-43 mainly includes cytoplasm construction of high phosphorylation TDP-43 and clearance of nuclear TDP-43 [1, 2, 7, 8].

2.8 Pathogenesis of ALS-related genes

The cellular processes, including RNA processing, protein degradation pathways, ubiquitin-proteasome system (UPS), autophagy, and so on, are all reported related to ALS pathogenesis [1–3, 7–22]. Sorted by the various processes, we summarize the causative genes and genes might increase susceptibility of ALS which impact physiological activities mentioned above (**Figure 1**).

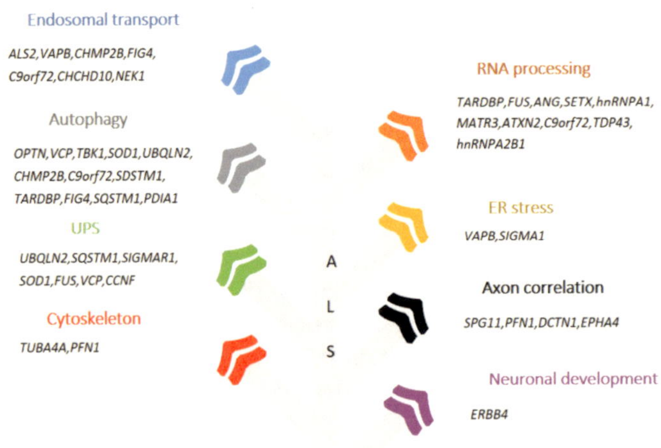

Figure 1.
Dysfunction cellular processes and related genes contributed to the pathogenesis of ALS.

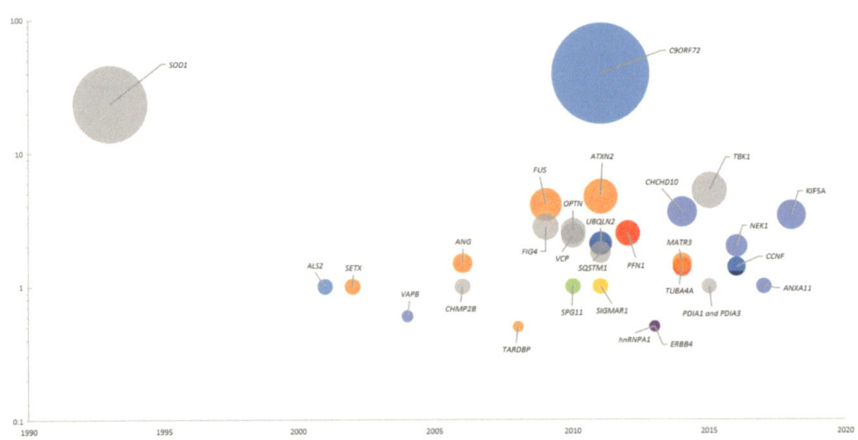

Figure 2.
The worldwide frequency of ALS-related genes. The x-axis is the time when genes discovered. The y-axis is the logarithms of the mutation frequency of genes in ALS. The mutation frequency of C9orf 72, CHCHD10, CCNF, KIF5A, and ANXA11 are only within FALS. Where gene frequency was not available (ALS2, SETX, SIGMAR1, and PDIA1), one "circle size" equivalent to 1% is given for illustrative purposes.

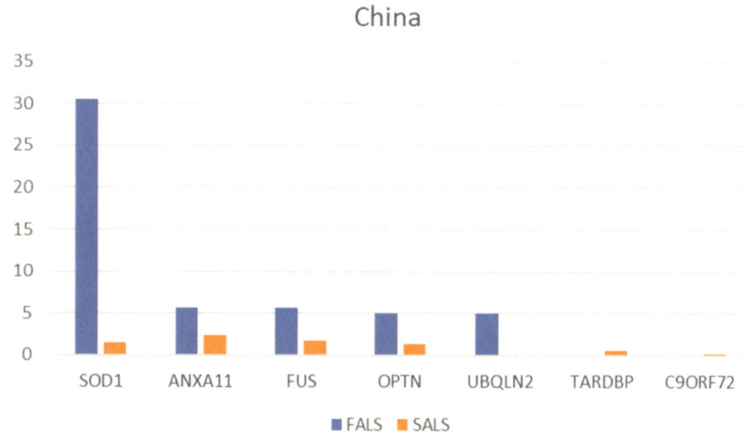

Figure 3.
ALS mutation genes frequency among FALS and SALS in Mainland China. The y-axis means the percentage of different mutation genes.

2.9 Advances on gene discovery and frequency

We describe the worldwide ALS distribution feature by frequency of occurrence in different regions (**Figure 2**) [1–3, 7–9, 11, 14, 23, 24]. We summarize ALS mutation genes frequency according to the researches in Mainland China (**Figure 3**).

3. GWAS on ALS

Recently, the studies on ALS have shown the development trend of the blowout with the technology improving, however, no longer limited by technical condition, the number of newly discovered ALS-related gene did not meet expectation. It indicates a shift in the genetic pathway that multiple genetic variants and environmental factors may interact simultaneously to increase ALS susceptibility. On the basis of the fact that sporadic form apparently accounts for high rate of ALS and the hypothesis that ALS may not appear to be familial in a conventional Mendelian manner, a new research method, genome-wide association study (GWAS), is applied to the research of ALS.

Since GWAS was applied to complex diseases, remarkable achievements have been made in certain fields. It is also hoped that in this way, we will be able to find the risk factors of ALS [25–27].

3.1 SNPs and GWAS

The International HapMap Project, which began in 2002, mapped the single-nucleotide polymorphisms (SNPs) haplotypes of the human genome from four major populations in the world and promoted the development of GWAS. At the same time, the rapid development of high-density and high-throughput genotyping technology, which can detect hundreds of thousands of SNPs in a single reaction, makes it possible to systematically screen mutations associated with complex diseases throughout the genome. Unlike previous candidate gene studies, GWAS does not need to build any assumptions based on disease pathophysiology prior to the study and can relatively be an unbiased screen for almost all common mutations in the genome. At present, some risk factors of complex diseases, such as age-related macular degeneration, diabetes mellitus, breast cancer, and so on, have been initially identified by GWAS.

3.2 ALS GWAS boot

Schymiek et al. firstly reported GWAS in SALS in February 2007 [28]. A total of 276 patients and 271 controls with white American ancestry were recruited in this research. They used a chip to detect 555,352 SNPs and found 34 of the most relevant SNPs by association analysis. For negative results, they elucidated that SALS might contain a group of diseases with similar clinical manifestations like FALS, each of which is determined by different mutation sites, and that different diseases and mutation sites may interfere with GWAS's shooting out of susceptible genes. Among the 34 SNPs, there was an overexpression of genes associated with cytoskeletal actin regulation. For example, the *KIAAl721* gene of rs11099864 and the *FMN2* gene of rs1037666 had a homologous region that played an important role in the regulation of cytoskeletal actin. The most closely related rs4363506 of 34 SNPs was located in the *DOCKl* gene, which plays an important role in nerve growth. Although no disease-susceptible gene was found, the study identified possible SNPs and published all the results, which facilitated subsequent large-scale SALS GWAS studies.

Recently, a series of ALS GWAS studies have been published and found several potential risk genes [29–32]. However, the results of these studies are different with the same ideas and methods. The biological process of some candidate genes is unclear, and the evidence needs to be supplemented.

4. Genetic testing

Gene testing helps ALS patients and families enhance their understanding on the condition and information requested in genotype-specific treatments. Although ALS patients desire access to genetic testing, genetic advances have been slow to reach the clinical care of the ALS patient. In recent years, the landscape of genetic testing and genetic counseling for ALS has been rapidly transformed with the identification of novel genes and the advent of next-generation sequencing technology.

4.1 Genetic testing options

As with all clinical testing, genetic risk assessment, including family history and pedigree analysis, and pretest counseling, helping patients anticipate the possible impact of genetic testing on themselves and their family members, are necessary for patients before genetic testing.

Currently available genetic testing options for ALS include Sanger sequencing for traditional simple mutations, assays for the *C9orf 72* repeat expansion, next-generation sequencing panels, whole-exome sequencing, and whole-genome sequencing.

4.2 Post-test counseling

Regarding the positive result, specific mutation, genotype-phenotype correlations, family history, and inheritance pattern should be thoroughly analyzed. Meanwhile, implications and risks for family members, including offspring and siblings, and theories about why the disease occurs also should be reviewed and addressed. For the reported definite pathogenic mutations, clinicians should provide information and hope about the potential genetic therapies in the future.

4.3 Presymptomatic testing

To increase certainty, make health or lifestyle choices, and make decisions about family planning, the presymptomatic testing could be conducted. According to the guidelines for presymptomatic genetic testing in other neurodegenerative diseases such as Huntington disease and Alzheimer disease, ALS should be tailored as following: pretest genetic counseling, baseline neurologic and cognitive assessment, psychological evaluation, in-person disclosure, presence of support person, and posttest genetic counseling. Most of important, presymptomatic testing should be offered to adult first-degree relatives of ALS patients with established mutations after written informed consent obtained [4].

5. Gene therapy

With the exception of riluzole, an anti-glutamatergic agent which was shown to prolong survival for 2–3 months by blocking the presynaptic release of glutamate, and edaravone, an antioxidant which was shown to decrease the rate of patient immobility, no effective treatment is currently available for ALS that can stop or reverse the disease progression.

Gene therapy is a promising therapeutic approach for ALS since it can be used to deliver "gene drugs," encoding for blocking the novel gene expression, antiapoptotic proteins, and for neurotrophic factors, to the motor neurons crossing the blood-brain barrier specifically to prevent further motor neuron degeneration and to preserve the function of remaining motor neurons.

Here, we are to illustrate some examples of each therapeutic strategy for describing the present status and advance of gene therapy treatment.

5.1 SOD1

The neurotoxicity of mutant SOD1 is related to the dose of the toxic protein through multiple pathological mechanisms. A potential therapeutic approach to SOD1-related ALS is to block the expression of the toxic SOD1 that could cause motor neuron degeneration [33]. This therapy option which is more worthy of attention is that it possibly avoids and decreases potential influence in downstream pathological cascades. Recently, the studies mostly focus on antisense oligonucleotides and RNA interference which are both to block gene expression through enhancing the degradation of RNA.

5.1.1 Antisense oligonucleotides in models and human

In animal models of *SOD1*-associated ALS, antisense oligonucleotide treatment significantly delayed disease onset, improved neuromuscular function, and prolonged survival.

The first clinical trial of antisense oligonucleotide treatment in human beings had favorable safety outcomes, and now the clinical trial to assess the safety, tolerability, and pharmacokinetics of a second generation SOD1 antisense oligonucleotide is in progress (Clinical Trials.Gov, NCT02623699) [34].

5.1.2 Short hairpin RNA (shRNA) treatment in mutant SOD1 ALS models

According to literature, in $SOD1^{G93A}$ mice, reduction of human *SOD1* expression can significantly slow ALS progression and extend survival by using a single peripheral injection of an adeno-associated virus serotype 9 (AAV9) encoding shRNA [35].

While, in a recent study reported, SOD1 expression in the motor cortex of P70 *SOD1*^{G93A} models was selectively silenced by delivery of AAV9-SOD1-shRNA. As a result, not only the ALS progression was slowed and the survival was extended significantly, but also the survival of spinal motor neurons was significantly enhanced [36].

5.1.3 miRNA treatment in mutant SOD1 ALS models and healthy nonhuman primates

In a study, scientists reported a new method that systemically delivered drug based on an artificial microRNA. In the *SOD1*^{G93A} mice, this drug delayed ALS onset, prolonged the survival, and significantly preserved muscle strength and motor and respiratory functions. Notably, the research of this drug has been conducted in nonhuman primates, and the result showed that *SOD1* expression in lower motor neurons was safely blocked [37].

5.2 C9orf72

Similar therapeutic approach targeting C9orf72 for ALS is also in development. The toxicity of mutated C9orf72 is imparted by the formation of nucleolar RNA foci that sequester important RNA-binding proteins and by the generation of toxic dipeptide repeat (DPR) proteins.

The C9orf72 hexanucleotide repeat expansion (HRE) of GGGGCC DNA and RNA enables the formation of complex structures including G-quadruplexes. Because the Guanosine-rich DNA and RNA sequences are prone to formation of G-quadruplexes, a stable four-stranded structure present within ribosomal DNA sequences, transcription start sites, the promoter and untranslated regions of mRNA, human telomeric DNA sequences. It may play an important role in various cellular processes such as telomere maintenance, ribosome biogenesis, gene replication, transcription, and translation. Therefore, both C9orf72 HRE DNA and RNA may contribute to the pathogenesis of ALS/FTD disease through a mechanism associated with their structure polymorphism. Presently, based on the above mechanism, two strategies including antisense-mediated interventions and small-molecule-based approach have been developed to interfere with neurodegenerative diseases associated with G-quadruplexes [38].

5.2.1 Antisense oligonucleotides in mutant C9orf72 ALS models

A recent study reported that the RNA foci and DPR proteins were reduced significantly in mutant C9orf72 ALS mice by a single-dose injection of antisense oligonucleotides to reduce C9orf72 RNA repeats, and after 6 months of treatment, the motor function was also preserved [39].

5.2.2 Small-molecule ligands targeting the G-quadruplex structure in mutant C9orf72 cells

The small-molecule ligands, such as porphyrin, acridine, pentacridium, telomestatin, naphthalene diamide, and bisquinolium, directly target and bind to the G-quadruplex structure and selectively modulated the function of the G-quadruplex. For example, TMPyP4, a cationic porphyrin, can bind and disrupt the secondary structures of C9orf72 HRE and even damage its interactions with hnRNPA1 and ASF/SF2 proteins [40].

Similarly, some studies also showed that three small-molecule ligands can bind G-quadruplex and decreased RNA foci and RNA translation in both cultured cells and patient-derived neurons [41].

5.3 Others

TBK1 is a key regulatory molecule upstream of OPTN, SQSTM1/p62, and IRF3 in the autophagy and neuroinflammatory pathways that are implicated in ALS. Manipulation of TBK1 might potentially compensate for defects caused by other ALS-associated proteins in these pathways—for example, VCP and UBQLN2. NEK1 and C21orf2 are known to interact at the protein level and, in addition to TUBA4A, PFN1, NEFH, and PRPH, they represent the building blocks of the cellular scaffold. Administration of small molecules that enhance cytoskeletal integrity could represent a viable therapy for stopping progression or reversing the disease course in patients with these mutations [4–6].

6. Conclusion

Nearly a decade ago, the only way to test ALS-related gene was SOD1 sequencing, whereas clinicians now have a wide availability of testing options already. Whole-exome sequencing is current standard in most related searches. However, the factors such as high rate of incomplete penetrance in ALS, few large pedigrees, and short survival of patients lead to the discovery of ALS-related genes worse than expected and the identification of susceptible mutations limited.

Although many known ALS-related genes' structural characteristics and roles have been discovered, which have highlighted critical processes, pathways, and intracellular localizations of dysregulation, there are still many reported variants with uncertain significance. Further functional studies are needed to clarify the pathogenesis of these genes. Till now, more people believe that ALS is the result of interaction between multiple genes that each increases the susceptibility of the disease, but does not initiate the pathogenesis alone. So, we need to do more research on oligogenic ALS cases. Most importantly, with the improvement of understanding of ALS genetics, we will have more opportunities to develop meaningful therapies.

Author details

Junling Wang
Department of Neurology, Xiangya Hospital, Central South University, Changsha, Hunan, China

*Address all correspondence to: wjling8002@126.com

References

[1] Recabarren-Leiva D, Alarcon M. New insights into the gene expression associated to amyotrophic lateral sclerosis. Life Science. 2018;**193**:110-123. DOI: 10.1016/j.lfs.2017.12.016

[2] Ghasemi M, Brown RJ. Genetics of amyotrophic lateral sclerosis. Cold Spring Harbor Perspectives in Medicine. 2018;**8**(5). DOI: 10.1101/cshperspect.a024125

[3] Volk AE, Weishaupt JH, Andersen PM, et al. Current knowledge and recent insights into the genetic basis of amyotrophic lateral sclerosis. Medizinische Genetik. 2018;**30**(2): 252-258. DOI: 10.1007/s11825-018-0185-3

[4] Roggenbuck J, Quick A, Kolb SJ. Genetic testing and genetic counseling for amyotrophic lateral sclerosis: An update for clinicians. Genetics in Medicine Official Journal of the American College of Medical Genetics. 2016;**19**(3):267

[5] Vajda A, Mclaughlin RL, Heverin M, et al. Genetic testing in ALS. Neurology. 2017;**88**(10):991-999

[6] Picher-Martel V, Valdmanis PN, Gould PV, et al. From animal models to human disease: A genetic approach for personalized medicine in ALS. Acta Neuropathologica Communications. 2016;**4**(1):70

[7] Chia R, Chiò A, Traynor BJ. Novel genes associated with amyotrophic lateral sclerosis: Diagnostic and clinical implications. Lancet Neurology. 2017;**17**(1)

[8] Al Sultan A, Waller R, Heath P, et al. The genetics of amyotrophic lateral sclerosis: Current insights. Degenerative Neurological & Neuromuscular Disease. 2016:**6**(1):49-64

[9] Maurel C, Dangoumau A, Marouillat S, et al. Causative genes in amyotrophic lateral sclerosis and protein degradation pathways: A link to neurodegeneration. Molecular Neurobiology. 2018; (Pt 2):1-20

[10] Woollacott IOC, Simon M. The C9ORF72 expansion mutation: Gene structure, phenotypic and diagnostic issues. Acta Neuropathologica. 2014;**127**(3):319-332

[11] Ticozzi N, Vance C, Leclerc AL, et al. Mutational analysis reveals the FUS homolog TAF15 as a candidate gene for familial amyotrophic lateral sclerosis. American Journal of Medical Genetics. Part B, Neuropsychiatric Genetics. 2011;**156B**(3):285-290. DOI: 10.1002/ajmg.b.31158

[12] Yuan Z, Jiao B, Hou L, et al. Mutation analysis of the TIA1 gene in Chinese patients with amyotrophic lateral sclerosis and frontotemporal dementia. Neurobiology of Aging. 2018:64

[13] Morgan S, Orrell RW. Pathogenesis of amyotrophic lateral sclerosis. British Medical Bulletin. 2016;**119**(1):87-98

[14] Yohei I, Masahisa K, Kensuke I, et al. Amyotrophic lateral sclerosis: An update on recent genetic insights. Journal of Neurology. 2013;**260**(11):2917-2927

[15] Ji AL, Zhang X, Chen WW, et al. Genetics insight into the amyotrophic lateral sclerosis/frontotemporal dementia spectrum. Journal of Medical Genetics, 2017;**54**(3):145-154

[16] Ajroud-Driss S, Siddique T. Sporadic and hereditary amyotrophic lateral sclerosis (ALS). Biochimica et Biophysica Acta. 2015;**1852**(4):679-684

[17] Chen S, Sayana P, Zhang X, Le W. Genetics of amyotrophic lateral

sclerosis: An update. Molecular Neurodegeneration. 2013;**8**(1):28

[18] Therrien M, Dion PA, Rouleau GA. ALS: Recent developments from genetics studies. Current Neurology & Neuroscience Reports. 2016;**16**(6):1-12

[19] White MA, Sreedharan J. Amyotrophic lateral sclerosis: Recent genetic highlights. Current Opinion in Neurology. 2016;**29**(5):557

[20] Norris FH, Sang UK, Denys EH, et al. Amyotrophic lateral sclerosis. The New England Journal of Medicine. 2017;**53**(8):162-172

[21] Corcia P, Couratier P, Blasco H, et al. Genetics of amyotrophic lateral sclerosis. La Presse Médicale. 2014;**43**(5):555-562

[22] Tripolszki K, Török D, Goudenège D, et al. High-throughput sequencing revealed a novel SETX mutation in a Hungarian patient with amyotrophic lateral sclerosis. Brain and Behavior: A Cognitive Neuroscience Perspective. 2017;**7**(4):e00669

[23] Smith BN, Topp SD, Fallini C, et al. Mutations in the vesicular trafficking protein annexin A11 are associated with amyotrophic lateral sclerosis. Science Translational Medicine. 2017;**9**(388):eaad9157

[24] Zhang K, Liu Q, Liu K, et al. ANXA11 mutations prevail in Chinese ALS patients with and without cognitive dementia. 2018;**4**(3):e237

[25] Ozaki K, Ohnishi Y, Iida A, et al. Functional SNPs in the lymphotoxin-alpha gene that are associated with susceptibility to myocardial infarction. Nature Genetics. 2002;**32**(4):650

[26] Klein RJ, Caroline Z, Chew EY, et al. Complement factor H polymorphism in age-related macular degeneration. Science. 2005;**308**(5720):385-389

[27] Macarthur J, Bowler E, Cerezo M, et al. The new NHGRI-EBI catalog of published genome-wide association studies (GWAS Catalog). Nucleic Acids Research. 2017;**45**(Database issue):D896-D901

[28] Schymick JC, Scholz SW, Fung H-C, et al. Genome-wide genotyping in amyotrophic lateral sclerosis and neurologically normal controls: First stage analysis and public release of data. The Lancet Neurology. 2007;**6**(4):291-292

[29] Travis D, Huentelman MJ, Craig DW, et al. Whole-genome analysis of sporadic amyotrophic lateral sclerosis. New England Journal of Medicine. 2007;**357**(8):775

[30] Michael A van ES, Paul WJ van Vught, Blawu HM, et al. Genetic variation in DPP6 is associated with susceptibility to amyotrophic lateral sclerosis. Nature Genetics. 2008;**40**(1):29-31

[31] Kawam AA, Alshawaqfeh M, Cai JJ, et al. Simulating variance heterogeneity in quantitative genome wide association studies. BMC Bioinformatics. 2018;**19**(Suppl 3):72

[32] Broce I, Karch CM, Wen N, et al. Immune-related genetic enrichment in frontotemporal dementia: An analysis of genome-wide association studies. PLoS Medicine. 2018;**15**(1):e1002487

[33] van Zundert B, Brown RH Jr. Silencing strategies for therapy of SOD1-mediated ALS. Neuroscience Letters. 2017;**636**:32-39

[34] Bishop KM. Progress and promise of antisense oligonucleotide therapeutics for central nervous system diseases. Neuropharmacology. 2017;**120**:56

[35] Foust KD, Salazar DL, Shibi L, et al. Therapeutic AAV9-mediated suppression of mutant SOD1 slows

disease progression and extends survival in models of inherited ALS. Molecular Therapy. 2013;**21**(12):2148-2159

[36] Thomsen GM, Gowing G, Latter J, et al. Delayed disease onset and extended survival in the SOD1G93A rat model of amyotrophic lateral sclerosis after suppression of mutant SOD1 in the motor cortex. Journal of Neuroscience the Official Journal of the Society for Neuroscience. 2014;**34**(47):15587

[37] Borel F, Gernoux G, Cardozo B, et al. Therapeutic rAAVrh10 mediated SOD1 silencing in adult SOD1(G93A) mice and nonhuman primates. Human Gene Therapy. 2016;**27**(1):19-31

[38] Kumar V, Kashav T, Islam A, et al. Structural insight into C9orf72 hexanucleotide repeat expansions: Towards new therapeutic targets in FTD-ALS. Neurochemistry International. 2016;**100**:11-20

[39] Jiang J, Zhu Q, Gendron T, et al. Gain of toxicity from ALS/FTD-linked repeat expansions in C9ORF72 is alleviated by antisense oligonucleotides targeting GGGGCC-containing RNAs. Neuron. 2016;**90**(3):535-550

[40] Zamiri B, Reddy K, Macgregor RB Jr, Pearson CE. TMPyP4 porphyrin distorts RNA G-quadruplex structures of the disease-associated r(GGGGCC)n repeat of the C9orf72 gene and blocks interaction of RNA-binding proteins. Journal of Biological Chemistry. 2014;**289**(8):4653-4659

[41] Su Z, Zhang Y, Gendron T, et al. Discovery of a biomarker and lead small molecules to target r(GGGGCC)-associated defects in c9FTD/ALS. Neuron. 2014;**83**(5):1043-1050

Chapter 6

Structural and Functional Consequences of the SMA-Linked Missense Mutations of the Survival Motor Neuron Protein: A Brief Update

Wei Li

Abstract

Genetically linked to the survival motor neuron 1 gene *SMN1*, spinal muscular atrophy (SMA) is an autosomal recessive neuromuscular disease with dysfunctional α-motor neurons. As the product of the *SMN1* gene, the survival motor neuron protein (SMN) plays an essential role in the molecular pathogenesis of SMA. On 1 June 2017, a PLoS ONE article reported a set of computational structural analysis to illustrate how do SMA-linked mutations of *SMN1* lead to structurally/functionally deficient variants of SMN. Following this article, this chapter provides a brief update of the structural and functional consequences of the missense mutations of this SMA protein.

Keywords: spinal muscular atrophy, survival motor neuron protein, missense mutation, structural consequence(s), functional consequence(s)

1. Setting the scene up

On 1 June 2017, *PLoS ONE* published an original research article (**Figure 1**) [1] with a title 'How do SMA-linked mutations of *SMN1* lead to structural/functional deficiency of the SMA protein?', of which this chapter aims to provide a brief update.

1.1 The genetics of SMA: a brief introduction

SMA is an autosomal recessive neuromuscular disease with α-motor neuron (anterior horn of the spinal cord) dysfunction and muscular atrophy [2]. SMA is caused by loss (~95% of SMA cases) or mutation (~5% of SMA cases) of the survival motor neuron gene 1 *SMN1* (telomeric *SMN*, *telSMN* or *SMN1*, GenBank: U18423, the 5q13 region of human chromosome) [3]. In the 5q13 region of the human chromosome, there is also a nearly identical *survival motor neuron 2* gene *SMN2* (centromeric *SMN*, *cenSMN* or *SMN2*, GenBank: NM_022875) [3]. The two genes (*SMN1* and *SMN2*) have been extensively characterised, and their roles in SMA have been reviewed in detail [2–8].

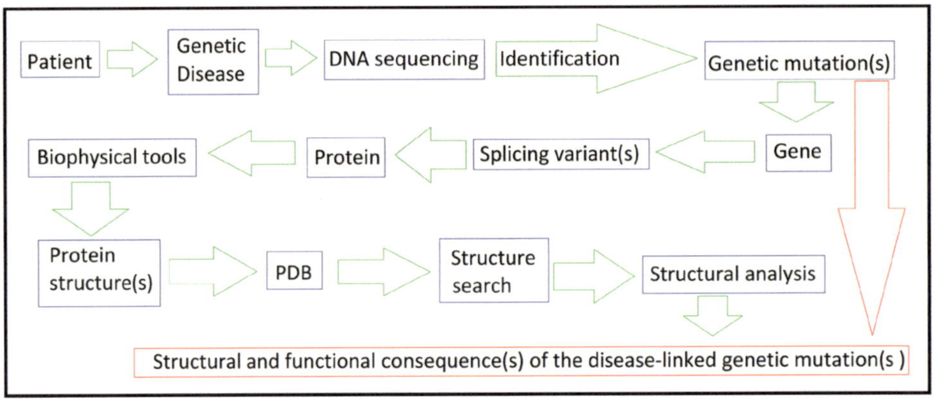

Figure 1.
A flow chart for the computational analysis of structural/functional consequences of clinically identified genetic diseases-linked missense mutation(s) of key gene(s) and protein(s). In [1], SMA was shown as an example of the computational analysis as illustrated here in this figure (http://biomedical-advances.org/ep-20182-14/).

1.2 The survival motor neuron protein and its role in SMA

The survival motor neuron (SMN) protein is the product of *SMN1*, the SMA-determining survival motor neuron gene [2, 3]. As a result, SMN is also called the SMA protein. In fact, the 38-kD SMN is the actually affected protein in SMA [9–11], and is a cytoplasmic protein that also occurs in dot-like nuclear structures called gems, which is why SMN is formerly termed Gemin1 [3, 12], too.

In the molecular pathogenesis of SMA, of particular interest is an exon 7-skipping splicing defect identified in the pre-mRNA editing of the *SMN2* gene [5]. Due to this splicing defect, *SMN2* predominantly produces exon 7-skipped transcripts, which encode a truncated isoform of the SMN protein (SMNΔ7 or SMN2 with 282 residues), in comparison with the full-length SMN protein with 294 residues (SMN1 or FL-SMN).

In pre-mRNA editing, spliceosome is the major functional unit, and spliceosomal small nuclear ribonucleoproteins (snRNPs) are essential components of the nuclear pre-mRNA processing machinery [13–17]. In the pathogenesis of SMA, the SMN protein plays a critical role in pre-mRNA processing, because the biogenesis of spliceosomal snRNPs is promoted by the SMN complex [14, 18, 19], which consists of SMN (Gemin1), Gemin2–8 and UNR-interacting protein (UNRIP) [13, 16, 20]. In the formation of the SMN complex, SMN forms oligomers and directly interacts via its N-terminus with Gemin2 and via its tudor domain with spliceosomal (Sm) proteins [13, 21, 22]. A key component of the SMN complex, SMN first assembles the essential SMN/Gemin complex, which in turn mediates the formation of the Sm core domain of the spliceosomal snRNPs [13, 21, 22].

2. Structural and functional consequences of the SMA-linked missense mutations of SMN

In general, genetic mutation includes missense, nonsense, insertion and deletion mutations. A nonsense mutation is a point mutation in a DNA sequence that results in a premature stop codon, or a nonsense codon in the transcribed mRNA, and in a truncated, incomplete and usually functionally deficient protein product. In contrast, a missense mutation involves substitution of one single amino acid residue, and therefore is able to provide unique access to residue-specific structural insights into the role of the residue in the structure and function of the target protein, provided that the three-dimensional structure of the target protein is experimentally determined and deposited in the Protein Data Bank. Thus, this chapter focuses on SMA-linked missense mutations of SMN and aims to provide a brief update of their structural and functional consequences with a set of computational structural analysis as described in [1].

2.1 An update of SMA-linked missense mutations of SMN

A set of point mutations (missense and nonsense mutations) have been previously summarised in [1], including A2G [23], nonsense mutation Q15X [24], D30N [25], D44V [25–27], V94G [28], G95R [25], Y130C [29], nonsense mutation Q157X [30], A188S [31], nonsense mutation W190X [32], nonsense mutation L228X [33], P245L [34], L260S [28], S262G and S262I [4, 25], M263T [32], S266P [29], Y272C [4, 35, 36], H273R [29], T274I [4, 35, 36], G275S [32], G279C and G279V [4, 35, 37, 38]. As of 25 September 2018, eight more missense mutations of SMN were summarised and reported, including A2V, Y109C, Y130C, Y130H, P221L, S230L, P244L and R288S [39].

2.2 An update of experimentally determined SMN-related structures

In [1], 11 SMN-related structures were retrieved from the PDB database [40] with 2 search parameters (text search for: survival motor neuron protein and molecule: survival motor neuron protein). In a new search of the PDB database (accessed 25 September 2018) [40] with the same parameters, 14 PDB entries were retrieved, including **1G5V**, **1MHN**, **2LEH**, **4A4E**, **4A4G**, **4GLI**, **4QQ6**, **4V98**, **5XJL**, **5XJQ**, **5XJR**, **5XJS**, **5XJT** and **5XJU**. In a comparison with the PDB entries in [1], during the past 16 months, six new SMN-related structures were deposited in the Protein Data Bank, including **5XJL** (to supersede **3S6N** [41]), **5XJQ** [42], **5XJR** [42], **5XJS** [42], **5XJT** [42] and **5XJU** [42]. While the six PDB entries do contain a set of different yet functionally related protein molecules, including snRNP Sm-D1, snRNP Sm-D2, snRNP E, snRNP F and snRNP G, they also contain a fragment of the survival motor neuron protein (SMN residues 26–62), according to the fasta format data of the six PDB entries [42].

2.3 An update of the structural and functional consequences of the missense mutations of SMN

2.3.1 Asp44 in the Gemin2-binding domain of SMN

In light of the six new experimentally determined SMN-related structures (**Table 1**), a new set of computational structural analysis, as previously described in detail in [1], is within the reach of this chapter to provide an update of it. Two aspartates (Asp 35 and Asp44) of SMN stood out in the structural analysis of both intramolecular and intermolecular salt bridges for this SMA protein, as listed in **Table 2**.

Asp44 is in the exon 2a of *SMN1* (the Gemin2-binding domain), and involved in an SMA-linked Asp44Val (D44V) missense mutation [25], which involves a substitution of Asp44's charged side chain by Val44's hydrophobic side chain. Of extraordinary functional significance is that SMN's Gemin2-binding activity is totally suppressed by the D44V mutation in *SMN1* [41]. Moreover, the D44V SMN (SMND44V) mutant's snRNP assembly activity is lower than that of the wild-type SMN (FL-SMN or SMN1) [27].

PDB ID	Structure title	Method	Release date
5XJL	Crystal structure of the Gemin2-binding domain of SMN, Gemin2 in complex with SmD1/D2/F/E/G from human	X-ray	2 May 2018
5XJQ	Crystal structure of the Gemin2-binding domain of SMN, Gemin2 in complex with SmD1(1–82)/D2/F/E/G from human	X-ray	4 July 2018
5XJR	Crystal structure of the Gemin2-binding domain of SMN, Gemin2dN39 in complex with SmD1(1-82)/D2/F/E/G from human	X-ray	4 July 2018
5XJS	Crystal structure of the Gemin2-binding domain of SMN, Gemin2dN39 in complex with SmD1(1-82)/D2/F/E from human	X-ray	4 July 2018
5XJT	Crystal structure of the Gemin2-binding domain of SMN, Gemin2 in complex with SmD1(1-82)/D2.R61A/F/E/G from human	X-ray	4 July 2018
5XJU	Crystal structure of the Gemin2-binding domain of SMN, Gemin2dN39 in complex with SmD1(1-82)/D2.R61A/F/E/G from human	X-ray	4 July 2018

In this table, X-ray represents X-ray crystallography as a biophysical tool for biomolecular structure determination.

Table 1.
A list of new (compared with those summarised in [1]) experimentally determined SMN-related structures as of 25 September 2018 [40].

In a solid alignment with the computational analysis in [1], a set of salt bridges were structurally identified between SMN's Asp44 (M_Asp_44) and Gemin2's Arg213 (2_Arg_213), as shown in **Table 2**. In particular, four intermolecular salt bridges were identified between the buried side chains (**Table 3**) of these two charged residues, i.e. according to the coordinates data in the PDB entry **5XJL** [42], as shown in **Figure 2**.

Taken together, it is conceivable that the buried side chains of SMN's Asp44 and Gemin2's Arg213 form a salt bridge, which constitutes a favourable electrostatic energy contribution to the SMN-Gemin2 complex structural stability [41], and highlights the functionally indispensable roles of the two residues' charged side chains, considering the experimental observation that the SMN-Gemin2 binding is abrogated by the D44V mutation [41], resulting in a functionally deficient SMA-linked D44V SMN mutant.

In addition to the intermolecular salt bridges formed between SMN's Asp44 and Gemin2's Arg213, a set of intramolecular salt bridges were also identified between side chains of SMN's Asp35 and Lys41 (**Table 2**), which was reported in [1], too, where 15 salt bridges were identified between the side chains of SMN's Asp35 and Lys41 in the salt bridge analysis of the NMR-determined SMN-Gemin2 complex ensemble (PDB ID: 2LEH) [22, 41]. In SMN, Lys41 is a positively charged residue and also a neighbouring residue of Asp44. Functionally different to the SMA-linked D44V mutation, a Lys41Ala (K41A) mutation (not SMA-linked) does not affect SMN-Gemin2 binding [41]. Thus, in another solid agreement with the structural analysis in [1], the structural analysis highlights that the salt bridges between SMN's Asp35 and Lys41 are intramolecular, i.e. within the apo SMN protein, instead of intermolecular, i.e. at the SMN-Gemin2 complex structure interface, which help to explain why the Lys41Ala (K41A) mutation is not SMA-linked [41].

Overall, there is a solid agreement between the old [1] and the new (this chapter) sets of computational structural analysis for both NMR and X-ray SMN-related structures, reflecting the technical maturity of the two main biophysical tools for biomolecular structure determination, particularly in light of the booming number of cryo-electron microscopy (cryo-EM) images uploaded to the Electron

PDB ID	SBnum	Residue A	Atom A	Residue B	Atom B	Distance (Å)
5XJL	4	M_ASP_44	OD1	2_ARG_213	NH1	2.946 (Yellow)
5XJL	4	M_ASP_44	OD1	2_ARG_213	NH2	3.579 (Red)
5XJL	4	M_ASP_44	OD2	2_ARG_213	NH1	3.236 (Brown)
5XJL	4	M_ASP_44	OD2	2_ARG_213	NH2	3.848 (Blue)
5XJQ	3	M_ASP_44	OD1	2_ARG_213	NH1	2.760
5XJQ	3	M_ASP_44	OD1	2_ARG_213	NH2	3.593
5XJQ	3	M_ASP_44	OD2	2_ARG_213	NH1	2.968
5XJR	2	M_ASP_44	OD1	2_ARG_213	NH1	2.385
5XJR	2	M_ASP_44	OD2	2_ARG_213	NH1	2.871
5XJS	3	M_ASP_44	OD1	2_ARG_213	NH1	3.078
5XJS	3	M_ASP_44	OD1	2_ARG_213	NH2	3.670
5XJS	3	M_ASP_44	OD2	2_ARG_213	NH1	2.631
5XJT	3	M_ASP_44	OD1	2_ARG_213	NH1	2.335
5XJT	3	M_ASP_44	OD1	2_ARG_213	NH2	3.386
5XJT	3	M_ASP_44	OD2	2_ARG_213	NH1	3.067
5XJU	2	M_ASP_44	OD1	2_ARG_213	NH1	2.302
5XJU	2	M_ASP_44	OD2	2_ARG_213	NH1	2.989
5XJQ	1	M_ASP_35	OD1	M_LYS_41	NZ	3.921
5XJS	2	M_ASP_35	OD1	M_LYS_41	NZ	3.670
5XJS	2	M_ASP_35	OD2	M_LYS_41	NZ	3.803
5XJT	2	M_ASP_35	OD1	M_LYS_41	NZ	2.416
XJT	2	M_ASP_35	OD2	M_LYS_41	NZ	2.931
5XJU	1	M_ASP_35	OD1	M_LYS_41	NZ	3.274

In this table, the residue naming scheme is **Chain ID_residue name_residue number,** *SBnum represents the number of salt bridges computationally identified from the PDB entries listed in this table. In the top four rows for PDB entry* **5XJL,** *Yellow, Red, Brown and Blue represent the colouring scheme for* **Figure 2**. *Distance represents the distance between two oppositely charged groups/atoms in Å.*

Table 2.
A summary of salt bridge analysis of the six new SMN-related structures as of 25 September 2018 [40].

Microscopy Data Bank (EMDB), where a long way is there to go still for cryo-EM to match NMR spectroscopy and X-ray crystallography in terms of technical maturity and the urgent need of tools for structural model quality validation [45].

2.3.2 Gly95 in the SMN tudor domain

Although not located in the structurally determined region of the six new structures (**Table 1**), Gly95 is a residue in the SMN tudor domain, and it is involved in a Gly95Arg (G95R) mutation [25]. This G95R mutation significantly reduces SMN's ability to bind Sm proteins, such as Sm-B and Sm-D1 [25], confirming that tudor domain is the essential binding site of SMN to Sm proteins.

In a further inspection of the computational analysis as reported in [1], no salt bridge or hydrogen bond was identified for Gly95. Nonetheless, in the SMN tudor domain NMR ensemble [46], between the side chains of Asp96 and Lys93, 1 salt bridge was found for PDB ID **1G5V** [46] with 10 structure models, 18 salt bridges

Residue	SASA (Å^2)	SASA-intrinsic (Å^2)	SASA-Ratio
2_Arg_213	57	238.76	0.238
M_Asp_44	67	140.39	0.477

In this table, SASA, SASA-intrinsic and SASA-ratio represent for SMN's Asp44 and Gemin2's Arg213 the average SASA value calculated by DSSP [43], the intrinsic SASA value [44] and the ratio of SASA divided by SASA-intrinsic, respectively. In this table, the residue naming scheme is **Chain ID_residue name_residue number**.

Table 3.
Solvent accessible surface area (SASA) values of SMN's Asp44 and Gemin2's Arg213 (PDB ID: **5XJL**) *[42].*

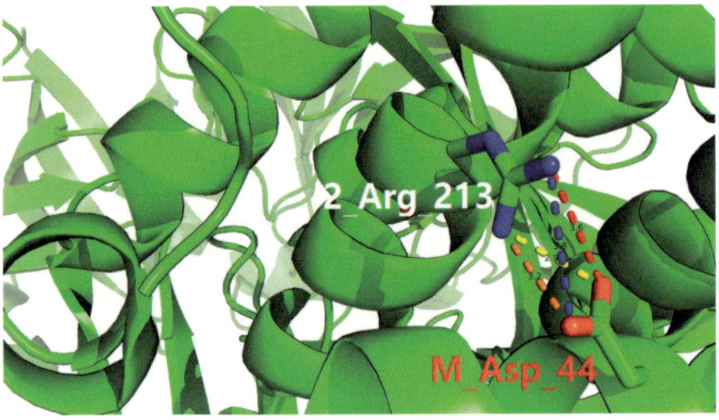

Figure 2.
Four salt bridges formed between the buried side chains of SMN's Asp44 (M_Asp_44 in red text) and Gemin2's Arg213 (2_Arg_213 in white text). In this figure, the residue naming scheme is **Chain ID_residue name_residue number**. *In this figure, Asp44's side chain oxygens are coloured red, and Arg213's nitrogen atoms are coloured blue, while all hydrogen atoms are coloured in white, the four dotted lines in four colours represent the four side chain salt bridges formed between the two oppositely charged residues, where the colouring scheme is described in* ***Table 2****.*

were found for PDB ID **4A4E** [47] with 20 structure models (**Figure 3**) and 16 salt bridges were found for PDB ID **4A4G** [47] with 20 structure models. Similarly, 15 salt bridges were also identified between the side chains of Glu147 and Lys97 of SMN (PDB ID: **4A4G** [47], with 20 structure models), with the distance between 2 oppositely charged groups being 2.93 ± 0.39 Å.

Quite interestingly, Gly95 sits right between the two oppositely charged neighbouring residues (Asp96 and Lys93), which are the only two charged residues in the

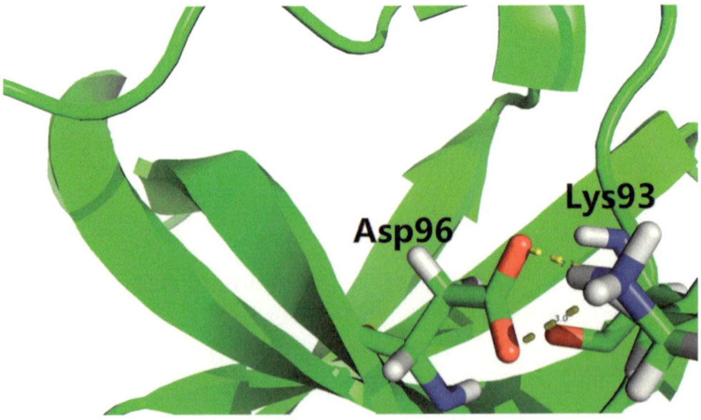

Figure 3.
Two salt bridges formed between the side chains of SMN's Asp96 and Lys93 (shown as sticks here) according to a salt bridge analysis of the third structural model of the NMR ensemble (PDB ID **4A4E***) [47]. In this figure, Asp96's side chain oxygens are coloured red, and Lys93's side chain nitrogen is coloured blue, while all hydrogen atoms are coloured in white.*

tudor domain that are in the spatial proximity of Gly95. Thus, it is conceivable that a G95R mutation disrupts the Asp96-Lys93 salt bridge and/or builds another one (possibly even stronger) between the side chains of Lys95 and Asp96, which either perturbs the structure-stabilising activity of the Asp96-Lys93 salt bridge, and/or makes it energetically more unfavourable for Asp96's side chain to orient towards positively charged side chains in Sm proteins and thereby affect the binding of SMN to Sm proteins. While the potential local electrostatic interaction disruption mechanism here for this SMA-linked G95R mutation is similar to that of the E134K and the Q136E mutations of SMN [1], the former mechanism is dependent on the occurrence of energetically unfavourable electrostatic interaction(s), but the latter mechanism is dependent on the loss of energetically favourable electrostatic interaction(s) for local structural stability of the SMN tudor domain, the essential part of SMN for the Sm protein-binding, which can help explain the reduced Sm core assembly activity of the two SMA-linked SMNE134K and SMNQ136E mutants.

2.3.3 Y109C, Y130C and Y130H in the SMN tudor domain

Among the eight SMN residues with SMA-linked missense mutations [39], only Y109 and Y130 are located in the structurally determined region of SMN [1], according to the updated list of SMN-related structures as of 25 September 2018. Although Y109C, Y130C and Y130H are not located in the structurally determined region of the six new structures, the three missense mutations are located in the structurally determined region of the experimentally determined structures [1].

Tyr130 is a tudor domain hydrophobic residue with a Tyr130Cys (Y130C) mutation [29]. In the computational analysis in [1], no salt bridge or hydrogen bond was identified for Tyr130. Nonetheless, Tyr130 is ~50% buried, with an *SASA* value of 111.1 ± 4.18 $Å^2$ compared with its standard *SASA* value at 212.7 $Å^2$, while Tyr109 is deeply buried, with an *SASA* value of 61.1 ± 8.43 $Å^2$ compared with its standard *SASA* value at 212.7 $Å^2$. Taken together, the *SASA* analysis of the three SMA-linked mutations highlights the potential significance of the deeply buried hydrophobic side chains of Tyr109 and Tyr130 in the SMN tudor domain.

PDB File	Acceptor (A)	Donor (D)	Hydrogen (H)	D-A (Å)	H-A (Å)	∠*ADH*(*)
0.pdb	OD2, A_ASP_105	OH, A_TYR_109	HH, A_TYR_109	2.73	1.80	13.75
3.pdb	OD2, A_ASP_105	OH, A_TYR_109	HH, A_TYR_109	2.69	1.77	15.61
4.pdb	OD2, A_ASP_105	OH, A_TYR_109	HH, A_TYR_109	2.67	1.72	10.96
5.pdb	OD2, A_ASP_105	OH, A_TYR_109	HH, A_TYR_109	2.77	1.86	17.26
6.pdb	OD2, A_ASP_105	OH, A_TYR_109	HH, A_TYR_109	2.71	1.78	15.09
8.pdb	OD2, A_ASP_105	OH, A_TYR_109	HH, A_TYR_109	2.78	1.87	16.14
12.pdb	OD2, A_ASP_105	OH, A_TYR_109	HH, A_TYR_109	2.83	1.95	20.70
14.pdb	OD2, A_ASP_105	OH, A_TYR_109	HH, A_TYR_109	2.71	1.78	13.76
18.pdb	OD2, A_ASP_105	OH, A_TYR_109	HH, A_TYR_109	2.71	1.76	10.91
19.pdb	OD2, A_ASP_105	OH, A_TYR_109	HH, A_TYR_109	2.63	1.70	13.36

In this table, the names of the PDB files correspond to the single NMR structural model split from the NMR ensemble (PDB entry **4A4E***) by a tcl script [1], the residue naming scheme is* **Chain ID_residue name_residue number***, ∠ADH represents the angle formed by acceptor (A), donor (D) and hydrogen (H) (∠ADH).*

Table 4.
The hydrogen bonds formed between the residue side chains between SMN's Tyr109 and Asp105 (PDB entry **4A4E***).*

What is more, in the computational analysis in [1], 10 side chain hydrogen bonds (**Table 4**) were identified between SMN's Tyr109 and Asp105 in the PDB entry **4A4E** [47], with the donor-acceptor distances (*D* - *A* in **Table 4**) at 2.72 ± 0.06 Å and ∠*ADH* at 14.75 ± 2.93, no salt bridge was identified for Asp105, and no further hydrogen bonds were identified for Tyr109 and Asp105 for all experimentally determined SMN-related structures as of 25 September 2018.

Taken together, the computational findings here indicate that SMN's Tyr109 and Asp105 contribute to the structural stability of SMN through hydrogen bonding between their side chains, as it is quite clear that if Tyr109 is replaced by Cys109, then the side chain hydrogen bond (**Figure 4**, **Table 4**) will disappear, and that the negatively charged side chain of Asp105 will gain more geometric freedom due to the disappearance of the hydrogen bond, which can cause a potential disruption of the (either intramolecular and/or intermolecular) electrostatic interaction network, not to mention the possibility of a disrupted disulphide bonding network within the SMN protein, the SMN complex or even the snRNP assembly, which is critical to ensure that pre-mRNA editing of the *SMN1* gene does not go wrong and that its product is the FL-SMN protein, instead of its truncated functionally deficient counterpart.

2.3.4 A structural analysis of the hydrogen bonds formed within the six new SMN-related structures

In light of the six new experimentally determined SMN-related structures (**Table 1**), a new set of hydrogen bonding analysis is conducted according to the details in [1], the result of which is briefly summarised in **Table 5**.

Table 5 shows the four hydrogen bonds formed between snRNP Sm-D2's Asp93 and Gemin2's Arg235 and Arg239. Functionally, Gemin2 is closely linked to SMN (formerly known as Gemin1), and NMR spectroscopy was used to experimentally determine a Gemin1-Gemin2 complex structure (PDB ID: 2LEH) [22, 41], making a closer visual inspection worthwhile of the SMN-related structures (PDB IDs: 5XJS, 5XJT and 5XJU [42], **Table 1**).

From **Figure 5** (PDB ID:5XJS), it is quite clear that the three charged residues (snRNP Sm-D2's Asp93 and Gemin2's Arg235 and Arg239) sit right at the structural interface between Sm-D2 (pink) and Gemin2 (green), with their oppositely

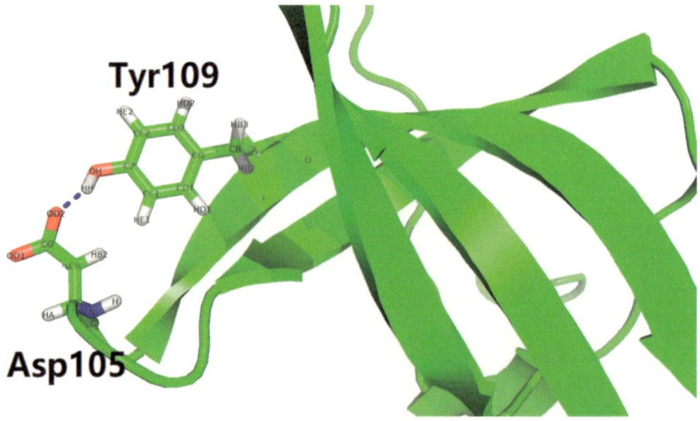

Figure 4.
*The hydrogen bond (**Table 4**) formed between the side chains of SMN's Tyr109 and Asp105 in the PDB entry **4A4E** [47]. In this figure, SMN's Tyr109 and Asp105 are shown in sticks, all side chain oxygens are coloured red, and side chain nitrogen is coloured blue, while all hydrogen atoms are coloured in white, and all atoms are labelled with their names nearby. The blue dotted line between OD2 of Asp105 and HH of Tyr109 represents the hydrogen bond formed between SMN's Tyr109 and Asp105.*

PDB ID	Acceptor (A)	Donor (D)	Hydrogen (H)	D-A (Å)	H-A (Å)	∠ADH(*)
5XJR	OE1, A_GLN_24	NH2, B_ARG_94	HH21, B_ARG_94	3.00	1.99	1.79
5XJR	OD2, B_ASP_104	NH1, B_ARG_102	HH12, B_ARG_102	2.98	2.07	20.93
5XJS	OD1, B_ASP_93	NE, 2_ARG_235	HE, 2_ARG_235	2.94	1.96	11.86
5XJS	OD1, B_ASP_93	NH2, 2_ARG_239	HH21, 2_ARG_239	2.98	1.98	5.80
5XJS	OD2, B_ASP_60	ND2, B_ASN_64	HD22, B_ASN_64	2.99	2.13	25.53
5XJT	OD1, B_ASP_93	NE, 2_ARG_235	HE, 2_ARG_235	2.65	1.75	21.43
5XJU	OD1, B_ASP_93	NE, 2_ARG_235	HE, 2_ARG_235	2.98	2.08	23.00
5XJU	OD2, B_ASP_60	ND2, B_ASN_64	HD21, B_ASN_64	2.80	1.99	29.63

In this table, the residue naming scheme is **Chain ID_residue name_residue number**, *∠ADH represents the angle formed by acceptor (A), donor (D) and hydrogen (H) (∠ADH).*

Table 5.
The hydrogen bonds formed between the residue side chains within the six new experimentally determined SMN-related structures.

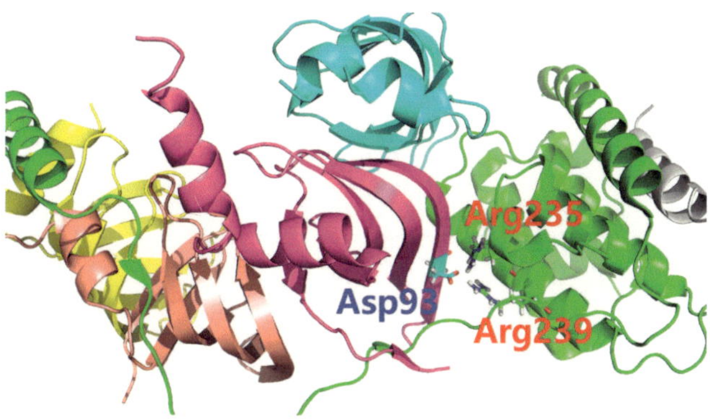

Figure 5.
Crystal structure of the Gemin2-binding domain of SMN, Gemin2 in complex with SmD1/D2/F/E (PDB ID: **5XJS** *[42]). In this figure, the whole structure is shown in cartoon and coloured by chain using PyMol [48], where green and pink represent Gemin2 and snRNP Sm-D2, respectively. In this figure, three amino acid residues are shown in sticks and labelled with red and blue texts nearby.*

charged side chains closely facing each other, similar to the situation as reported by [1], where the deeply buried side chains of SMN's Lys45 and Asp36 act as two electrostatic clips at the SMN-Gemin2 interface via interactions with both the side chains and the backbone of Gemin2's Gln105, Gln109, His120, His123 and Trp124.

In the subsequent computational salt bridge analysis of the six new SMN-related structures, it turned out that the three charged residues did form salt bridges between their closely facing oppositely charged side chains, as listed in **Table 6** below and illustrated in **Figure 6**.

Collectively, snRNP Sm-D2's Asp93 and Gemin2's Arg235 and Arg239 are three structurally important residues which help stabilise the structural interface through intermolecular electrostatic interactions, including both salt bridges and also hydrogen bonds, similar to the way SMN's Asp44, Gemin2's Arg213 and the two SMN residues (Lys45 and Asp36) play stabilising roles in the SMN-Gemin2 complex structure formation [1].

Considering the intimate functional relationship between Gemin2 and SMN, a further set of structural analysis was conducted for the hydrogen bond and the salt bridge for Arg235 and Arg239 of PDB entry 2LEH [22, 41], and it turned out that

PDB ID	SBnum	Residue A	Atom A	Residue B	Atom B	Distance (Å)
5XJL	3	B_ASP_93	OD1	2_ARG_239	NH1	3.734
5XJL	3	B_ASP_93	OD1	2_ARG_239	NH2	3.052
5XJL	3	B_ASP_93	OD2	2_ARG_239	NH2	3.052
5XJQ	3	B_ASP_93	OD1	2_ARG_239	NH1	3.817
5XJQ	3	B_ASP_93	OD1	2_ARG_239	NH2	3.059
5XJQ	3	B_ASP_93	OD2	2_ARG_239	NH2	3.004
5XJR	3	B_ASP_93	OD1	2_ARG_239	NH1	3.811
5XJR	3	B_ASP_93	OD1	2_ARG_239	NH2	3.022
5XJR	3	B_ASP_93	OD2	2_ARG_239	NH2	2.938
5XJS	3	B_ASP_93	OD1	2_ARG_239	NH1	3.688
5XJS	3	B_ASP_93	OD1	2_ARG_239	NH2	2.983
5XJS	3	B_ASP_93	OD2	2_ARG_239	NH2	3.092
5XJT	2	B_ASP_93	OD1	2_ARG_239	NH2	3.251
5XJT	2	B_ASP_93	OD2	2_ARG_239	NH2	3.163
5XJU	3	B_ASP_93	OD1	2_ARG_239	NH1	3.634
5XJU	3	B_ASP_93	OD1	2_ARG_239	NH2	3.084
5XJU	3	B_ASP_93	OD2	2_ARG_239	NH2	3.089
5XJL	2	B_ASP_93	OD1	2_ARG_235	NH2	3.657
5XJL	2	B_ASP_93	OD2	2_ARG_235	NH2	3.475
5XJQ	2	B_ASP_93	OD1	2_ARG_235	NH2	3.686
5XJQ	2	B_ASP_93	OD2	2_ARG_235	NH2	3.647
5XJR	2	B_ASP_93	OD1	2_ARG_235	NH2	3.847
5XJR	2	B_ASP_93	OD2	2_ARG_235	NH2	3.800
5XJS	2	B_ASP_93	OD1	2_ARG_235	NH2	3.548
5XJS	2	B_ASP_93	OD2	2_ARG_235	NH2	3.379
5XJT	2	B_ASP_93	OD1	2_ARG_235	NH2	3.258
5XJT	2	B_ASP_93	OD2	2_ARG_235	NH2	3.766
5XJU	1	B_ASP_93	OD1	2_ARG_235	NH2	3.996

In this table, the residue naming scheme is **Chain ID_residue name_residue number,** *SBnum represents the number of salt bridges computationally identified from the PDB entries listed in this table. Distance represents the distance between two oppositely charged groups/atoms in Å.*

Table 6.
A summary of salt bridge analysis of the six new SMN-related structures as of 25 September 2018 [40].

the two arginines did not form any intermolecular electrostatic interaction with SMN, neither salt bridge nor hydrogen bond. Instead, the 2 arginines of Gemin2 only formed 2 hydrogen bonds with Gln272 and His231 of Gemin2, and 1 stable salt bridge with Asp274 of Gemin2, where 16 salt bridges were identified for the 32 NMR structural models (**Table 7**), according to the structural analysis of PDB entry **2LEH** [22, 41].

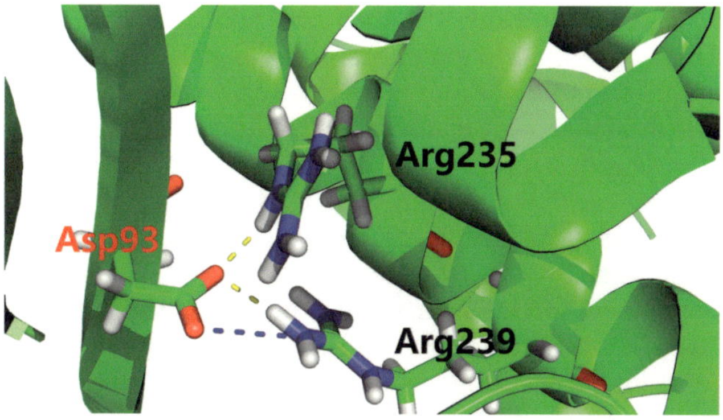

Figure 6.
Crystal structure of the Gemin2-binding domain of SMN, Gemin2 in complex with SmD1/D2/F/E (PDB ID: **5XJS***) [42]. In this figure, the yellow dotted lines represent two examples of the hydrogen bonds formed between Asp93 and Arg235, while the blue dotted line represents an example of the salt bridge formed between Asp93 and Arg239 (***Table 6***).*

PDB ID	SBnum	Residue A	Atom A	Residue B	Atom B	Distance (Å)
24.pdb	2	A_ASP_274	OD1	A_ARG_239	NH2	3.797
24.pdb	2	A_ASP_274	OD2	A_ARG_239	NH2	2.738
01.pdb	1	A_ASP_274	OD2	A_ARG_235	NH2	3.577
02.pdb	1	A_ASP_274	OD2	A_ARG_235	NH2	3.164
04.pdb	1	A_ASP_274	OD2	A_ARG_235	NH2	3.195
09.pdb	1	A_ASP_274	OD2	A_ARG_235	NH2	2.692
16.pdb	1	A_ASP_274	OD2	A_ARG_235	NH1	3.871
17.pdb	1	A_ASP_274	OD2	A_ARG_235	NH1	2.868
19.pdb	1	A_ASP_274	OD2	A_ARG_235	NH1	3.718
21.pdb	2	A_ASP_274	OD2	A_ARG_235	NH1	3.457
21.pdb	2	A_ASP_274	OD2	A_ARG_235	NH2	3.429
23.pdb	1	A_ASP_274	OD2	A_ARG_235	NH2	3.798
24.pdb	1	A_ASP_274	OD2	A_ARG_235	NH2	2.888
26.pdb	3	A_ASP_274	OD1	A_ARG_235	NH2	3.770
26.pdb	3	A_ASP_274	OD2	A_ARG_235	NH1	3.836
26.pdb	3	A_ASP_274	OD2	A_ARG_235	NH2	2.442
31.pdb	1	A_ASP_274	OD2	A_ARG_235	NH2	3.403

In this table, the residue naming scheme is **Chain ID_residue name_residue number***, SBnum represents the number of salt bridges computationally identified.*

Table 7.
A summary of salt bridge analysis of PDB entry 2LEH [22, 41].

3. Concluding remarks

Given SMN's critical role in the maturation of snRNP and in the development of SMA [2, 6, 11], it is necessary for the structure-activity relationship (SAR) characterisation to continue for the SMA protein. With various biophysical tools available for structural determination, for SMN-related proteins and biological complexes, such as the SMN complex and snRNPs, their structure determination and functional characterisation will undoubtedly continue to advance, which will be helpful both in further understanding of SMN's role in SMA from a molecular structural point of view. In practice, however, advancements do not come easy. For instance, although both full-length structures of FL-SMN (with 294 residues) and SMNΔ7 (with 282 residues) were already experimentally determined using X-ray crystallography and deposited in the database (PDB IDs: 4NL6 and 4NL7), they were subsequently withdrawn by the author because the sample used for the structure determination was wrong. Otherwise, these two full-length SMN structures would constitute the very first step towards a comprehensive picture of the structural and functional insights into SMN's role in the molecular pathogenesis SMA.

As of 25 September 2018, there is still no full-length SMN (or the SMN complex or the snRNP assembly) structure deposited in the wwPDB website [40], although it contains six new experimentally determined SMN-related structures, in addition to those reported in [1]. In terms of amino acid sequence, those SMN-related structures are still only SMN fragments, ranging from Gly26 to Lys51, and from Asn84 to Glu147. In between, there is still structurally not-determined-yet regions (referred to as **structural gaps** below) consisting of 204 SMN residues. Sixteen months have passed since the publication of [1], the structural gaps still remain, literally zero progress has been made to bridge them in spite of the six newly deposited structures, calling **again** [1] for further comprehensive structural determination and functional research for this SMA protein.

4. A residue-specific distributional analysis of the structural gaps in the Protein Data Bank

As a 38-kD protein, SMN is essentially a small one in terms of molecular weight, in comparison with all proteins whose structures have been deposited in the Protein Data Bank (PDB), a primary database for experimentally determined structures of biological molecules [40]. As discussed above, even for a protein as small as SMN, experimental structure determination does not seem simple or easy, especially when it has to be done in a full-length and gapless manner. Therefore, to test whether any residue-specific statistical pattern (not known yet before this chapter) exists in the structural gaps in the whole Protein Data Bank (accessed 25 September 2018), this chapter presents a set of residue-specific distributional analysis of all structural gaps throughout PDB.

While the number of experimentally determined protein structures keeps increasing in the PDB, with the number of cryo-EM structures [49] on the rise, X-ray crystallography and NMR spectroscopy remain to date the two main (**Table 8**) supplementary biophysical tools in structural biology, both with strengths and weaknesses [50, 51].

In PDB-format data, the atomic coordinates presented in ATOM records in a PDB file may not exactly match the sequence in the SEQRES records. However, these amino acids will often be included in the SEQRES records, since the portion of the chain was present during the experiment. In these cases, a 'REMARK 465' entry will be included in the header of the PDB file to identify each missing residue. For X-ray crystallography data, the ends of chains and mobile loops are often not observed in crystallographic experiments, and as a result, atomic coordinates are not included as ATOM records in the file, leading to the occurrence of gaps for structure determined by X-ray crystallography. Among currently available biophysical tools, NMR spectroscopy is able to provide unique access to atomic-level structural dynamic behaviour of protein molecules in solution under physiological conditions (such as temperature, pH, etc.). As a result, this chapter focuses on

Experimental method	Proteins	Nucleic acids	Protein/NA complex	Other	Total
X-ray	121,081	1958	6257	10	129,306
NMR	10,848	1256	250	8	12,362
Electron microscopy	1750	31	623	0	2404
Other	244	4	6	13	267
Multi-method	117	5	2	1	125

Table 8.
A summary of the number of experimentally determined biomolecular structures in PDB as of 25 September 2018.

the structural gaps within protein structures determined by NMR spectroscopy, and aims to test whether any residue-specific statistical pattern exists in them. Here, structural gaps are defined as protein fragments with residues which exist in the originally studied molecule as shown in the SEQRES records, but not in the observed structure/atomic coordinates.

As of 20 September 2018, 10,844 NMR-determined protein structures have been deposited in the Protein Data Bank, according to a structure search with two parameters (molecule type = protein, experimental method = NMR). After the 10,844 PDB files were downloaded from the PDB website, the numbers of the total and the missing amino acid residues were extracted with an in-house python script for all proteins, as listed in **Table 9**.

Residue	Missing no.	Total no.	Ratio = Missing no./Total no.
A	1782	75,627	0.023
C	152	25,777	0.00589673
E	1811	79,729	0.022
D	1390	59,908	0.023
G	3321	81,347	0.041
F	615	38,993	0.015
I	640	55,070	0.011
H	5146	26,182	0.196
K	1442	75,766	0.019
M	1203	23,652	0.050
L	1439	90,833	0.015
N	831	43,080	0.019
Q	1273	44,594	0.028
P	1518	46,205	0.032
S	3159	73,904	0.042
R	1234	52,761	0.023
T	1112	56,787	0.019
W	138	13,211	0.010
V	980	70,252	0.013
Y	626	32,905	0.019
Sum	29,812	1,066,583	0.027

Table 9.
The numbers of the total and the missing amino acid residues in NMR-determined protein structures as of 25 September 2018.

In total, the 10,844 protein structures contains 1,066,583 amino acid residues, ~2.8% of which (29812) are missing, i.e. the atomic positions of the 29,841 residues were not experimentally determined by NMR spectroscopy, although they were present in the NMR sample during the structural determination process.

From **Figure 7**, it can be seen that for 19 residues (excluding histidine), the missing ratio is well below or pretty close to 5%, while the missing ratio is 19.6% for histidine, as shown by the blue sharp peak on **Figure 7**. In a statistical one sample t-test analysis of the 19 missing ratios, it turned out 100% acceptable (P=1) that the average of ratio is 0.0231, and that the fitness between the 19 missing ratios and the red horizontal line (**Figure 8**) is 100% acceptable (P=1), according to a statistical Chi-square test, as revealed by **Figure 8**.

While a missing ratio of 5% might be considered statistically insignificant, a missing ratio of 19.6% is clearly not to be ignored here, raising one obvious question: what on earth is so special about histidine that makes it so special among the 20 naturally occurring amino acids in this residue-specific distributional analysis of the structural gaps?

Similar to the other 19, histidine is a naturally occurring amino acid that is used in the biosynthesis of proteins. Also similar to the other 19, it contains an amino group (which is in the protonated —NH3+ form under biological conditions) and a carboxylic acid group (which is in the deprotonated —COO^- form under biological conditions). In particular, histidine has an imidazole side chain (which is partially protonated), classifying it as a positively charged amino acid at physiological pH (~7.4). That is, among the 20 naturally occurring amino acids, five (Arg, Lys, His, Glu and Asp) possess ionisable side chains. Among the five, histidine is the only one whose side chain has an ionisable (with an intrinsic pKa at 6.04) [52, 53] imidazole ring structure, which can exist in two inter-convertible tautomeric states. While at a pH of 7.0, the imidazole ring is mostly deprotonated (proton occupancy = 9.88%), at a pH of 6.0, the imidazole ring is largely protonated (proton

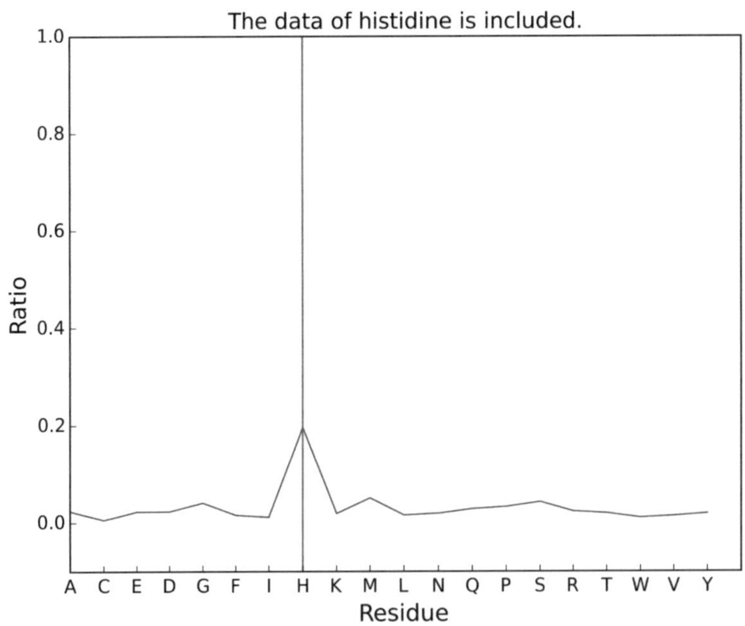

Figure 7.
A residue-specific distribution of the missing residues in NMR-determined protein structures as of 25 September 2018. In this figure, x-axis represents the one-letter codes for amino acid residues, and y-axis represents the residue-specific ratio of missing versus total residues in those NMR structures. The red vertical line highlights histidine as a particular residue with an outstanding missing ratio.

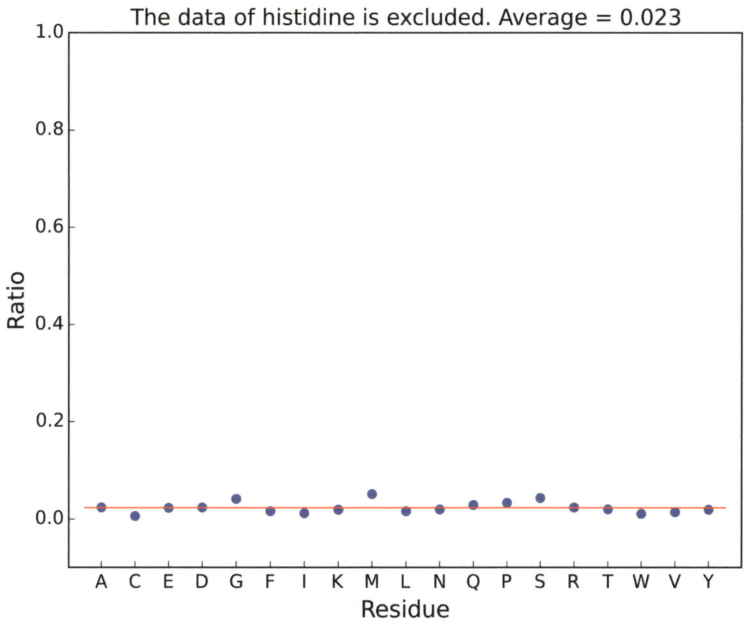

Figure 8.
A residue-specific scatter plot of the missing residues in NMR-determined protein structures as of 25 September 2018. In this figure, x-axis represents the one-letter codes for amino acid residues, and y-axis represents the residue-specific ratio of missing versus total residues in those NMR structures. The red horizontal line represents the average missing ratio level of the 19 residues.

occupancy = 52.30%), as defined by the classical Henderson-Hasselbalch equation [50], where the positively charged imidazole ring bears two NH bonds and has a positive electric charge, which is equally distributed between both nitrogens. As the pH increases, the imidazole ring loses the positive charge, and the remaining proton of the neutral imidazole ring can reside on either nitrogen, giving rise to two tautomeric states of the histidine side chain [52, 54, 55].

To sum up, it is probable that the missing ratio of histidine is much higher than the other 19 because it has a special side chain with special dynamic structural and physicochemical properties (such as stacking interaction [56]), and with a special imidazole ring in constant protonation-deprotonation equilibrium [57] and two tautomeric states [52, 54, 55], making its NMR-observables (chemical shift for instance) difficult to be experimentally observed and measured by NMR spectroscopy and structurally calculated by NMR-related software in the structural determination of proteins. To address this issue of PDB-wide structural gaps, selective isotope labelling of histidine residues (the side chains in particular) can be a useful approach in biomolecular structural determination by NMR spectroscopy, not just alone, but also in collaboration with other biophysical tools, not just for the special histidine, but also for its 19 siblings in the fundamental building block of life.

Author details

Wei Li
Institute of Nautical Medicine, Nantong University, Nantong City, Jiangsu Province, China P. R.

*Address all correspondence to: liweiqidong@stu.edu.cn

References

[1] Li W. How do SMA-linked mutations of SMN1 lead to structural/functional deficiency of the SMA protein? PLoS One. 2017;**12**(6):e0178519

[2] Burghes AHM. When is a deletion not a deletion? When it is converted. American Journal of Human Genetics. 1997;**61**(1):9-15

[3] Lefebvre S, Bürglen L, Reboullet S, Clermont O, Burlet P, Viollet L, et al. Identification and characterization of a spinal muscular atrophy-determining gene. Cell. 1995;**80**(1):155-165

[4] Lorson CL, Strasswimmer J, Yao JM, Baleja JD, Hahnen E, Wirth B, et al. SMN oligomerization defect correlates with spinal muscular atrophy severity. Nature Genetics. 1998;**19**(1):63-66

[5] Hua Y, Vickers TA, Okunola HL, Bennett CF, Krainer AR. Antisense masking of an hnRNP A1/A2 intronic splicing silencer corrects SMN2 splicing in transgenic mice. American Journal of Human Genetics. 2008;**82**(4):834-848

[6] Burghes AH, Beattie CE. Spinal muscular atrophy: Why do low levels of survival motor neuron protein make motor neurons sick? Nature Reviews Neuroscience. 2009;**10**(8):597-609

[7] Hua Y, Sahashi K, Hung G, Rigo F, Passini MA, Bennett CF, et al. Antisense correction of SMN2 splicing in the CNS rescues necrosis in a type III SMA mouse model. Genes & Development. 2010;**24**(15):1634-6144

[8] Hua Y, Sahashi K, Rigo F, Hung G, Horev G, Bennett CF, et al. Peripheral SMN restoration is essential for long-term rescue of a severe spinal muscular atrophy mouse model. Nature. 2011;**478**(7367):123-216

[9] Liu Q, Dreyfuss G. A novel nuclear structure containing the survival of motor neurons protein. EMBO Journal. 1996;**15**(14):3555-3565

[10] Carvalho T, Fcalapez AA, Lafarga M, Berciano M, Carmo FM. The spinal muscular atrophy disease gene product, SMN: A link between snRNP biogenesis and the Cajal (coiled) body. Journal of Cell Biology. 1999;**147**(4):715-727

[11] Young PJ, Le TT, Dunckley M, Nguyen TM, Burghes AH, Morris GE. Nuclear gems and Cajal (coiled) bodies in fetal tissues: Nucleolar distribution of the spinal muscular atrophy protein, SMN. Experimental Cell Research. 2001;**265**(2):252-261

[12] Young P, Ntlorson MC, Le T, Androphy E, Burghes A, Morris G. The exon 2b region of the spinal muscular atrophy protein, SMN, is involved in self-association and SIP1 binding. Human Molecular Genetics. 2000;**9**(19):2869-8277

[13] Seng CO, Magee C, Young PJ, Lorson CL, Allen JP. The SMN structure reveals its crucial role in snRNP assembly. Human Molecular Genetics. 2015;**24**(8):2138-2146

[14] Grimm C, Chari A, Pelz JP, Kuper J, Kisker C, Diederichs K, et al. Structural basis of assembly chaperone-mediated snRNP formation. Molecular Cell. 2013;**49**(4):692-703

[15] Pellizzoni L, Charroux B, Dreyfuss G. SMN mutants of spinal muscular atrophy patients are defective in binding to snRNP proteins. Proceedings of the National Academy of Sciences. 1999;**96**(20):11167-11172

[16] Pellizzoni L. Essential role for the SMN complex in the specificity of snRNP assembly. Science. 2002;**298**(5599):1775-1779

[17] Workman E, Saieva L, Carrel TL, Crawford TO, Liu D, Lutz C, et al. A

SMN missense mutation complements SMN2 restoring snRNPs and rescuing SMA mice. Human Molecular Genetics. 2009;**18**(12):2215-2229

[18] Otter S, Grimmler M, Neuenkirchen N, Chari A, Sickmann A, Fischer U. A comprehensive interaction map of the human survival of motor neuron (SMN) complex. Journal of Biological Chemistry. 2007;**282**(8):5825-8533

[19] Chari A, Golas MM, Klingenhäger M, Neuenkirchen N, Sander B, Englbrecht C, et al. An assembly chaperone collaborates with the SMN complex to generate spliceosomal SnRNPs. Cell. 2008;**135**(3):497-509

[20] Gubitz AK, Feng W, Dreyfuss G. The SMN complex. Experimental Cell Research. 2004;**296**(1):51-56

[21] Liu Q, Fischer U, Wang F, Dreyfuss G. The spinal muscular atrophy disease gene product, SMN, and its associated protein {SIP1} are in a complex with spliceosomal snRNP proteins. Cell. 1997;**90**(6):1013-1021

[22] Sarachan KL, Valentine KG, Gupta K, Moorman VR, Gledhill JM, Bernens M, et al. Solution structure of the core SMN-Gemin2 complex. Biochemical Journal. 2012;**445**(3):361-370

[23] Monani UR, Pastore MT, Gavrilina TO, Jablonka S, Le TT, Andreassi C, et al. A transgene carrying an A2G missense mutation in the SMN gene modulates phenotypic severity in mice with severe (type I) spinal muscular atrophy. Journal of Cell Biology. 2003;**160**(1):41-52

[24] Wirth B. An update of the mutation spectrum of the survival motor neuron gene *SMN1* in autosomal recessive spinal muscular atrophy (SMA). Human Mutation. 2000;**15**(3):228-237

[25] Sun Y, Grimmler M, Schwarzer V, Schoenen F, Fischer U, Wirth B. Molecular and functional analysis of intragenic SMN1 mutations in patients with spinal muscular atrophy. Human Mutation. 2005;**25**(1):64-71

[26] Zhang ML, Lorson CL, Androphy EJ, Zhou J. An in vivo reporter system for measuring increased inclusion of exon 7 in SMN2 mRNA: Potential therapy of SMA. Gene Therapy. 2001;**8**(20):1532-1538

[27] Ogawa C, Usui K, Aoki M, Ito F, Itoh M, Kai C, et al. Gemin2 plays an important role in stabilizing the survival of motor neuron complex. Journal of Biological Chemistry. 2007;**282**(15):11122-11134

[28] Clermont O, Burlet P, Benit P, Chanterau D, Saugier Veber P, Munnich A, et al. Molecular analysis of SMA patients without homozygous SMN1 deletions using a new strategy for identification of SMN1 subtle mutations. Human Mutation. 2004;**24**(5):417-427

[29] Prior TW. Spinal muscular atrophy diagnostics. Journal of Child Neurology. 2007;**22**(8):952-956

[30] Brichta L, Garbes L, Jedrzejowska M. Nonsense-mediated messenger RNA decay of survival motor neuron 1 causes spinal muscular atrophy. Human Genetics. 2008;**123**(2):141-153

[31] Zapletalová E, Hedvičáková P, Kozák L, Vondráček P, Gaillyová R, Maři'ková T, et al. Analysis of point mutations in the SMN1 gene in SMA patients bearing a single SMN1 copy. Neuromuscular Disorders. 2007;**17**(6):476-481

[32] Alías L, Bernal S, Fuentes-Prior P, Barceló MJ, Also E, Martínez-Hernández R, et al. Mutation update of spinal muscular atrophy in Spain: Molecular characterization of 745 unrelated patients and identification of four novel mutations in the SMN1 gene. Human Genetics. 2008;**125**(1):29-39

[33] Tsai C, Jong Y, Hu C, Chen C, Shih M, Chang C, et al. Molecular analysis of SMN, NAIP and P44 genes of SMA patients and their families. Journal of the Neurological Sciences. 2001;**190**(2):35-40

[34] Rochette CF, Surh LC, Ray PN, Mcandrew PE, Prior TW, Burghes AHM, et al. Molecular diagnosis of non-deletion SMA patients using quantitative PCR of SMN exon 7. Neurogenetics. 1997;**1**(2):141-147

[35] Shpargel KB, Gall JG. Gemin proteins are required for efficient assembly of Sm-class ribonucleoproteins. Proceedings of the National Academy of Sciences of the United States of America. 2005;**102**(48):17372-73717

[36] Hahnen E, Schönling J, Rudnik-Schöneborn S, Raschke H, Zerres K, Wirth B. Missense mutations in exon 6 of the survival motor neuron gene in patients with spinal muscular atrophy (SMA). Human Molecular Genetics. 1997;**6**(5):821-285

[37] Talbot K, Ponting CP, Theodosiou AM, Rodrigues NR, Surtees R, Mountford R, et al. Missense mutation clustering in the survival motor neuron gene: A role for a conserved tyrosine and glycine rich region of the protein in RNA metabolism? Human Molecular Genetics. 1997;**6**(3):497-500

[38] Wang CH, Papendick BD, Bruinsma P, Day JK. Identification of a novel missense mutation of the SMN^T gene in two siblings with spinal muscular atrophy. Neurogenetics. 1998;**1**(4):273-276

[39] Sneha P, Zenith TU, Habib USA, Evangeline J, Kumar DT, Doss CGP, et al. Impact of missense mutations in survival motor neuron protein (SMN1) leading to spinal muscular atrophy (SMA): A computational approach. Metabolic Brain Disease. 2018:1-12. https://link.springer.com/article/10.1007%2Fs11011-018-0285-4

[40] Berman H, Henrick K, Nakamura H. Announcing the worldwide protein data bank. Nature Structural Biology. 2003;**10**(12):980

[41] Zhang R, So BR, Li P, Yong J, Glisovic T, Wan L, et al. Structure of a key intermediate of the SMN complex reveals Gemin2's crucial function in snRNP assembly. Cell. 2011;**146**(3):384-395

[42] Yi ZRH. Structures of 7S mutant complexes. Available from: http://wwwrcsborg/structure/5XJQ [to be published]

[43] Kabsch W, Sander C. Dictionary of protein secondary structure: Pattern recognition of hydrogenbonded and geometrical features. Biopolymers. 1983;**22**(12):2577-2637

[44] Hubbard SJ, Thornton JM. Naccess. Computer Program. Vol. 2. London: Department of Biochemistry and Molecular Biology, University College London; 1993

[45] Baker M. Cryo-electron microscopy shapes up. Nature. 2018;**561**(7724):565-567

[46] Sattler M, Selenko P, Sprangers R, Stier G, Bühler D, Fischer U. SMN tudor domain structure and its interaction with the Sm proteins. Nature Structural Biology. 2001;**8**(1):27-31

[47] Tripsianes K, Madl T, Machyna M, Fessas D, Englbrecht C, Fischer U, et al. Structural basis for dimethylarginine recognition by the tudor domains of human SMN and SPF30 proteins. Nature Structural & Molecular Biology. 2011;**18**(12):1414-1420

[48] DeLano WL. Pymol: An open-source molecular graphics tool. CCP4 Newsletter On Protein Crystallography. 2002;**40**:82-92

[49] Wu J, Yan Z, Li Z, Qian X, Lu S, Dong M, et al. Structure of the voltage-gated calcium channel $Ca_V1.1$ at 3.6 Å resolution. Nature. 2016;**537**(7619):191-196

[50] Li W. Gravity-driven pH adjustment for site-specific protein pKa measurement by solution-state NMR. Measurement Science and Technology. 2017;**28**(12):127002

[51] Li W. NMR-observed atomic bond length stability supports a dimensionality shift in protein main chain 3D structure description and representation. Current Research Bioorganic and Organic Chemistry. 2018;**2018**(2):1-4

[52] Pelton JG, Torchia DA, Meadow ND, Roseman S. Tautomeric states of the active-site histidines of phosphorylated and unphosphorylated IIIGlc, a signal-transducing protein from *Escherichia coli*, using two-dimensional heteronuclear NMR techniques. Protein Science. 2008;**2**(4):543-558

[53] Hansen AL, Kay LE. Measurement of histidine pKa values and tautomer populations in invisible protein states. Proceedings of the National Academy of Sciences. 2014;**111**(17):E1705-E1712

[54] Li S, Hong M. Protonation, tautomerization, and rotameric structure of histidine: A comprehensive study by magic-angle-spinning solid-state NMR. Journal of the American Chemical Society. 2011;**133**(5):1534-1544

[55] Wolff N. Histidine pKa shifts and changes of tautomeric states induced by the binding of gallium-protoporphyrin IX in the hemophore HasASM. Protein Science. 2002;**11**(4):757-765

[56] Wang L, Sun N, Terzyan S, Zhang X, Benson DR. A histidine/tryptophan π-stacking interaction stabilizes the heme-independent folding core of microsomal apocytochrome b5 relative to that of mitochondrial apocytochrome b5. Biochemistry. 2006;**45**(46):13750-13759

[57] Hass MAS, Yilmaz A, Christensen HEM, Led JJ. Histidine side-chain dynamics and protonation monitored by 13C CPMG NMR relaxation dispersion. Journal of Biomolecular NMR. 2009;**44**(4):225-233